Tremulous Prism

Our Journey in Dementia

A Memoir by Christopher Keith

This story is a factual memoir.

Photos and cover images are property of the author.

Tremulous Prism: Our Journey in Dementia

Copyright © 2015 Christopher Keith

ISBN: 978-1511861601

Quahog Press

Blue Hill, Maine

www.tremulousprism.wordpress.com

To the memory of Stephen and Barbara Keith

"Through a tremulous prism, I distinguish the features of relatives and familiars, mute lips serenely moving in forgotten speech."

Vladimir Nabokov

from *Speak, Memory* (1951)

CONTENTS

Preface ix

My Grandmother's Pair of Shears 1

Florida Sunshine 5

Skin 7

Yellow Jackets 11

Boat Building River 15

Morning Hours 19

Publisher's Clearinghouse 23

Persistent Thoughts 27

Nevermore 35

Card Games 43

Eye Drops 49

Pain Pills 55

Modern Times 59

Wedding Rings 71

Dignity Network 77

A Good Nail 79

War Medals 91

Dad 97

Where to Live 107

Voices 115

Swallow Studies 125

Halloween, Thanksgiving and Christmas 133

Pithlachascotee River 151

Reflection 155

About the Author 163

PREFACE

---◆---

Tremulous Prism

I borrow the title from a passage from the linguistic genius, Vladimir Nabokov, a brilliant man who loved life and family. Nabokov used the phrase "tremulous prism" to describe the many-faceted, distorted view of people and places we have as we look far back through the years.

This story describes recent family events related to the passing of my mother and father, events that mark the end of a generation. I want to record some of the scenes and conversations that show the concerns of old people facing certain decline, scenes that depict them battling in their last hours under circumstances that none of us anticipated. I want to share these impressions before they ultimately meld into the prismatic realm of things remembered.

MY GRANDMOTHER'S PAIR OF SHEARS

———— ⬥ ————

Yّears before I considered moving in with my parents, years before my parents became confused and needy of help, my grandmother, Rena Moore, had "gone crazy."

We called her "Grammie Moore." She had been a dedicated mother and a productive worker her entire life, working as a seamstress at Needleman's store on Main Street in Newport, Vermont. I recall feeling sorry for Grammie Moore when I was a child because she was born on February 29, Leap Year, and had only a handful of actual birthdays.

During my first two years in high school, our family lived in Newport along with both sets of my grandparents, maternal and paternal, although Grammie Moore's husband died of a heart attack when my mother was twenty-one. I never met him.

I sometimes felt guilty walking past her apartment on Second Street, knowing that she deserved a visit, knowing that I spent more time on School Street at my paternal grandparents, the Keiths.

She was a gentle, loving woman. At a certain point, though, she was unable to live by herself in her apartment. Her son, my uncle Charles, took her into his house halfway up Vance Hill Road in Newport Center.

On Vance Hill Road, Grammie Moore had a view of Lake Memphremagog which was nothing short of spectacular. She had the company of Charles and his wife, Dolores, and she had the pleasure of frequent visits from her grandchildren, Barbara Ann, Johnnie, David, and Terry and their spouses.

But none of that mattered. Grammie Moore was intractable. Difficult. For some reason, she didn't like living on Vance Hill, despite the view, despite the visits, despite family.

Grammie Moore went into a group home in Newport not far from the Cathedral of the Sacred Heart.

One Christmas, I picked her up in Newport and drove her up to Montreal in my father's black Thunderbird. As we drove north along Lake Memphremagog, we mentioned the names of the landmarks we could see out the car window: Mt. Orford, Owl's Head, Bear Mountain, Jay Peak. Grammie Moore repeated those names nonstop all the way to Montreal, whether or not there was a mountain within view. I was glad to give her a ride, but the repetitions of all those words made me wonder about her.

When we got to my parents' townhouse in Pointe Claire, we opened Grammie Moore's suitcase and found several pairs of eyeglasses within it, including pairs of men's eyeglasses. Grammie Moore had picked up random pairs of glasses belonging to other residents of the boarding house where she stayed in Newport and had packed them in her suitcase.

I had hoped that those residents didn't have to read any small print that Christmas weekend.

As her dementia progressed, my grandmother was placed in a nursing home in Newport. The following year, I visited her there just before Thanksgiving.

It was a cool, dark day. I had spent the morning at my paternal grandparents' house, the Keiths, raking leaves and creating huge piles of leaves shaped like burial mounds.

I stopped at Spates' greenhouse and bought a yellow rosebud in a little vase for Grammie Moore.

"I'm here to visit Rena Moore," I told the receptionist.

"She's in the common room," the receptionist said.

I expected to walk into a zoo full of elderly people, but that was not the case. I found my grandmother sitting in a wheelchair, staring into space, alone in the large common room. I looked around at the couches that were unoccupied, the fireplace that was unlit, the television that was not playing. Crystals of snow beat against the large panes of glass meeting the wind off Lake Memphremagog.

I gave the rosebud to Grammie Moore, and she touched it. I'd thought she might refuse it or throw it on the floor.

She used my name when she addressed me.

"Christopher," she said. "Don't ever have children. It hurts too much when you have to be away from them."

I didn't know what to say. I felt sorry that Grammie Moore had come to such a conclusion.

She looked across the room and called to "Charlie," her son, as if he were there with us.

We chatted for a little while. When I got up to leave, I said, "I hope you're okay, Grammie."

"When I wear black," she said.

At the door to the lobby, I looked back at her. She was examining the yellow rosebud.

A few days later, she got out a pair of scissors and cut her bedroom linen into strips. She cut up the sheet, the pillowcase, the curtains.

A lifelong seamstress, my grandmother had lashed out in the manner that was hers. She had raged against her incarceration and her dementia, and I was proud of her.

This act of rage, though, resulted in Grammie Moore being held down with bed restraints. Restraints kill the spirit and hasten a person's physical decline. The next time my mother drove from Montreal to Newport to visit Grammie Moore, she found the bed in Grammie Moore's room stripped and empty. She hadn't gotten the news that her mother had died.

FLORIDA SUNSHINE

I magine a person becoming eccentric and difficult to the point that even family members hesitate to be around them. Imagine a loved one who no longer relates to us as loved ones ordinarily do—with openness and generosity. A person with dementia exists in a world quite foreign to us. They may exhibit new preoccupations and fears, concerns and compulsions that we never saw in them up to this point. Even if they do become fearful and strange, we can still decide how we wish to treat *them*.

Many of us don't have to imagine a parent or spouse experiencing dementia. We can recall the onset of our loved one's confusion and the episodes that sealed the diagnosis. We saw the deterioration of our loved ones' coping skills and their transformation of personality from someone of inestimable closeness to us into people we hardly knew, people living a non-rational existence.

We've met each other, the surviving children and other caretakers, within screened porches of nursing homes and on tiled floors outside our loved ones' rooms in the rehab centers. Where we come from doesn't matter. The same dilemma strikes us. How best to care for them? How much of ourselves can we give? We may begin the conversation as strangers, yet as we speak openly about the experience and gain access to the emotion, we can find comfort and inspiration in the experience of another. We are brought closer together by the magnitude of the need on both sides—our own need and the person with dementia's.

Regardless of the size of the house, the degree of comfort it offers, the types of trees outside, the weather patterns, the regional accent—the onset of dementia can force the loved one out of their home into the starker environment of an institution. Those of us who visit them and care for them are unified in compassion, bound by a thread of hope, drawn to each other by the hint of any creative solution.

A creative solution to the predicament of needing to give, needing to understand, and to give and understand without exhausting oneself.

SKIN

—•◈•—

Barbara had pale freckled skin, delicate skin, skin that bruised easily as a result of her years of Prednisone use. When Barbara bumped into objects, her skin tore like tissue paper. Besides getting wounded accidentally, her skin underwent many procedures to remove patches of melanoma. The dermatologist, Dr. Monticiollo, aggressively removed lesions and biopsied all suspicious tissue, sending Barbara home with gauze bandages on her face, arms, legs. More wounds accrued before the last ones could heal. The appointments wore Barbara out with interminable waiting time in a johnny in an ice-cold office, the cutting of the tissue and the stitching of the skin grafts, the long healing process leading to follow-up visits. I sympathized with her because I had the same dermatologist.

At a yard sale that I held after my parents had passed away, Barbara's well-stocked first aid kit was the first item to go.

It was a blue, soft plastic box containing three pairs of scissors, several rolls of surgical tape, plenty of Band-Aids and boxes of gauze patches. The CNA who bought the kit had left her car running, popped open the trunk of the car, and scampered up the driveway. She rifled through a deep cardboard box and found the first aid kit like she knew it was there, like she could smell it.

My parents were Stephen and Barbara Keith, a couple approaching their sixtieth marriage anniversary. My decision to move to Florida and live with my parents had been long in the making, but I was jarred into action by Barbara sharing the results of a PET scan indicating hot spots for melanoma in her armpit, throat and breast.

They'd been telling neighbors for a year that one of their children was bound to come down to Florida to "help" them. Still, I had the feeling that my move was an attempt to achieve the impossible, the unthinkable. Two years would pass before I was convinced that I had made the right decision.

I was comfortable in my parents' pleasant home in Tall Pines at River Ridge on the corner of Baltusrol and Pineneedles Drive, having stayed in one of their guest bedrooms during many Christmas holiday visits. For me, the shock factor developed out of uprooting myself from a stable environment in Portland, Maine, and gambling on the success of this possibly awkward and emotional venture.

As it turned out, I was given a reprieve of sorts at the end of my first week living in Florida. Stephen and Barbara took a trip to Bow Lake in Strafford, New Hampshire, to visit their youngest daughter, Joanna, and her husband, John. I relaxed at 10435 Pineneedles Drive, watched *Shark Week* on television, and tried to get organized for school. I'd gotten a part-time job teaching English Comp at a nearby community college. While Stephen and Barbara were away, though, I received unsettling news from my dermatologist in Maine. He had biopsied a cracked, unhealed blemish on my nose, and the report indicated a basal cell carcinoma.

Ironically, Barbara's latest PET scan showed that all her hot spots had subsided. That left me as the one who had to schedule a Mohs procedure while Barbara was in the clear again.

After their trip, Stephen and Barbara arrived safely at Tampa International where I met them and drove them back home. Glad to get out of the humid dog days of New England, they entered their cool living room and collapsed in their chairs, declaring their trip the "last time" they would ever go on vacation.

I had missed them while they were away. I missed the unassuming little couple who inhabited the stucco house with its high ceilings and glass doors and trusty air conditioner. They described their pleasure in taking a boat ride with Joanna and John, the quiet beauty of Bow Lake, the loons swimming with their young, an excursion like a last echo of their many motorboat trips up Lake Memphremagog in Vermont, trips taken when they were middle-aged and healthy and their children were visiting.

Barbara had the pale, freckled skin of a redhead, a young beauty who had attended Syracuse University for one semester. Her father, Walter Moore, had suddenly died before the start of Barbara's second semester. She couldn't bear the thought of her mother living by herself, so she quit school and went back home to Newport, Vermont, to work as a telephone operator. There, she married my father, her high school classmate but a year younger.

Barbara was now an attractive, white-haired lady in her early eighties, somewhat hunched over but well dressed and aptly accessorized, who drove herself to the hair dresser every Wednesday afternoon. She drove both to her appointments and to Stephen's. He could no longer drive because he had lost vision in his good eye due to a herpes Zoster infection.

At a time when Barbara's vision was dull and blurry, she underwent cataract surgery at St. Luke's Eye Center. Following the surgery, her eyesight cleared up, but she was shocked and disappointed when she looked into the vanity mirror and her face came into focus, her soft facial skin creased with innumerable wrinkles.

YELLOW JACKETS

I came to the front of the house where Barbara was tending to her flower bed. She wore crinkled pants, a long-sleeved shirt, a hat, sunglasses, and flowered garden gloves. She was stooped over, straight-legged, pulling dead plants from the mulch, piling them on a white plastic bag laid out on the grass.

All through the hot sunlit air, dozens of yellow jackets flew about her faster than atoms in a circuit. They coursed the yard in near-swarm density over the flower garden and hedge and around the corner of the house. They were F-16 fighter-sized yellow jackets, Africanized, I thought, although they were probably the usual, huge Florida yellow jackets.

"I can't do much work for very long," Barbara said. "I don't have it in me anymore."

"Aren't there a lot of bees out here?" I said.

"They don't bother you if you don't pay any attention to them," she said.

Barbara kept working. The front entrance to the house was flanked by two Sago palms, a male palm topped with a mushroom of spores and one female. The log edger around the mulched flower bed was stained with mildew and nearly buried in the turf of the lawn. The yellow jackets were so thick it was like looking through a screen.

In sixteen years of visiting this house, I had never seen such an infestation. Barbara may have been able to live and let live with yellow jackets, but I was not. Sooner or later we would need a Realtor to show this property, and someone cruising the subdivisions looking at curb appeal wouldn't be impressed. The flying hoard of elongated black dots would put off anyone in their right mind. This couldn't be ignored.

Barbara went inside to rest. After making plans to change out all the stained blocks of log edger around the flower bed and deciding to kill the yellow jackets, I too went inside. It was three o'clock. Stephen was taking his daily drink of VO mixed with Diet Canada Dry ginger ale. I joined him in the living room with a beer in my hand as the first Rhodes piano chords of the theme to *Law & Order* were struck.

I sat down on the couch. I wasn't sure whether Stephen saw my presence as the companionship of a loyal son or as an intrusion on his afternoon. I suspected the latter. He did not acknowledge me with a nod or a hello, but he lifted his drink, which Barbara had mixed, took a sip and gave no indication as to whether he liked it.

Judge Judy always played on the TV set following the re-run of *Law & Order*. Stephen watched the judge berate her plaintiffs and defendants while Barbara nodded out in her recliner, her pencil falling between the cushions and the book of word puzzles sliding off her legs.

After supper, the front lawn was in shadow. I found the yellow jacket nest behind the azalea hedge, its dark, round opening in the sandy soil like the bore of an elephant gun. Aiming the black cone of the insecticide bomb at the opening, I gave the nest a long blast of poison and then mounded soil on it and tamped it down. Then I sped into the safety of the garage.

The next day, the air in our yard was completely free of yellow jackets.

A lady in a nearly subdivision had not been as lucky. The eighty year-old lady had tripped and fallen out in the middle of her lawn, angering a nest of yellow jackets. They swarmed from the ground and engulfed her, stinging her arms, face, invading her clothing, yet she had flailed and fought them, and doctors later said that her flailing had helped save her. Luckily, just as she lay engulfed in the swarm of yellow jackets, her son had arrived at the house and came running to pull her to safety.

In the ER, nurses shaved her head bald because bees kept pouring out of her hair.

I followed this story on the evening news. The newscaster speculated that alarm pheromones had incited the entire nest of yellow jackets to attack. The yellow jackets had injected the lady with so much poison that the serums the doctors gave her were not working. She didn't have the metabolism to clear the poisons out of her system. The TV news broadcast showed the family standing by the lady's hospital bed, staring at imminent death. The lady's life hung in the balance for a month, yet somehow she pulled through. The last I heard of her, she was still feeble, but she was on her way home.

BOAT BUILDING RIVER

T he Pithlachascotee River scrolls through clump-grass prairie, pine flats and palmetto forest on its way to the Gulf of Mexico, coursing through "old" New Port Richey, broadening into Millers Bayou, a choppy expanse of shining blue water. In the powerful sea breezes of autumn, people gather in open-air bars along the bayou to drink frozen margaritas and watch Tampa Bay Buccaneers football and observe the Hooters girls changing shifts.

Local families fish off the landing docks in Simms Park, where the Cotee River river slides under the Main Street bridge, and metalwork letters on the edifice of the bridge have been altered to read "New Pot Richey."

There are some nice homes along the river, their spacious yards stretching down to boat lifts on the riverbank, the houses shaded by a growth of pine trees, Washingtonia palm and cedar. The downtown is quaint and empty except for a pair of motorcycles throbbing abreast down a stretch of Grand Boulevard. At the corner of Grand and Nebraska Avenue stands the Richey Suncoast Theatre—whose early benefactors included Marilyn Monroe—the theatre a stucco art deco treasure whose cool interior hides a cast rehearsing *Li'l Abner*.

Spreading east from the Gulf and U.S. Route 19, though, you find neighborhoods of ranch style homes, low duplexes and triplexes fighting the smudge of mildew, chained dogs guarding properties without lawn irrigation, blighted palms that have never been fertilized, car ports packed with rusted barbeque grills, planters, urns, statues, lawn mowers in disrepair, and other clutter.

A mile inland, Massachusetts Avenue runs easterly to a stretch called Decubellis Road, formerly Moon Lake Road, renamed for his own family by Dave Decubellis, a county road and bridge superintendent.

There, the Pithlachascotee River narrows. Even its name ("boat building river" in Creek) is smaller, foreshortened to Cotee on the signage of a local elementary school. Across Little Road, the sod companies, self-storage units and multi-bay garages along Decubellis thin out. Ponds emerge, and fields are cut at intervals by sandy lanes that lead back into the oaks.

At night, Decubellis Road is well-tracked by coon and armadillo. By day its seething tar is crossed by rat snake and black racer, its gutters kept free of flesh by crow and vulture. In the heat of daylight, vultures crowd and hop on the carcass of a doe with the animation of a television nature special. Down the road, more of them shock the unwary traveler by pulling apart in mid-air the body of a black and white cat.

The Cotee is only a strand where it traces the northwest corner of the 8,000 acre Starkey Wilderness Preserve—a saw palmetto cradle to cottonmouth, turkey and boar. Starkey Park abuts River Ridge Golf Course, and together these lush properties wrap around Hunt Ridge, a prim subdivision where Stephen and Barbara Keith lived.

My mother and father moved to the Hunt Ridge development following their third year of retirement. They bought the model home on Lot 1, Hunt Ridge Unit 11, Tall Pines at River Ridge, in 1992, with my sister Alison as agent, that being the only transaction of her real estate career: 10435 Pineneedles Drive. Not long after the Keiths took up residence, the subdivision filled in with houses, the whippoorwills fled, the sod of the lawns took hold, and the methodical routines of many late middle-aged residents were confirmed.

Years passed, cocooned under a blue sky, the palm fronds gently rustling. The rampant development of Pasco County, Florida, could be ignored. The only challenges to the sleepy quietude of the neighborhood were the cry of the red-shouldered hawk and the squawk of the red-bellied woodpecker.

By the year 2000, the age restriction on the subdivision was extinguished. Older residents passed away, their homes purchased by younger families. Renters—undesirables—occupied certain of the houses, and the compulsive throttling of motorcycles shook the still morning.

MORNING HOURS

B efore dawn, the laboring whine of the trash compactor alerts us that it is morning and our obligations are once again upon us, then stillness descends and we can sleep for a while longer.

Later, Stephen Keith opens the door to the master bedroom and crosses the living room. His steps are careful, his motions haltingly deliberate. He wears short pants, moccasin-style loafers and an unzipped blue windbreaker. His swarthy skin is visible beneath gray chest hair.

Stephen pulls the cords of the window blinds. The blinds raise with the sound of a deck of cards being shuffled. One ripple follows another until the blinds on the three windows are raised halfway. In the view from the dining area, the Sago palms spread stiffly, and the trunk of a queen palm rises past the window casing.

Across the street, the solid, waxy foliage of a magnolia tree blocks the view of a neighbor's fig tree, while to the other side a red maple stands shaded with black like a carefully planned piece of photo realism.

Stephen's fingers trace the top rail of a chair at the dining room table as he passes into the living room, extending his arm as he shuffles by the closed panels of an outmoded Hitchcock entertainment center. The pastel portraits of his three daughters reign from the wall high above the couch.

He tugs a cord to open the set of vertical, white cloth blinds on the glass doors behind his wife's recliner chair.

To follow are the wide folded blinds in the arch of windows at the glass table where they eat all their meals and where Barbara reads the paper to Stephen each morning. Light floods through the rounded quadrant of the glass table top, streams over the white kitchen counter and across the white-tiled floor of the kitchen.

Next in line, the vertical blinds on the sliding door to the Florida room are drawn out of the way, creaking.

The burglar bar and the small locks on the door click apart. The door rumbles open. Stephen steps onto the ceramic tiles of the Florida room, his fingers pointed ahead as if he is going to touch someone on the arm and tell them his story. He shuffles to the far side of the room where eight orchids—all phalaenopsis—are snuggled into white wicker jardinières.

Plastic frames shriek as Stephen inches open only two of the many panels of vinyl windows.

Later on, by four-thirty or five o'clock at the latest, Stephen will close all the blinds again as if performing a funereal rite, entombing the house in shade despite the sparkle and caress of Florida's afternoon sunshine.

Stephen unlocks the door to the garage and presses a button to activate the garage door opener. He crosses the garage and goes out into the surprisingly cool morning air. Cardinals are whistling and rustling in the hedge. A Carolina wren investigates an azalea. Stephen retrieves the rubber garbage can and lid from the end of the driveway and picks up the newspaper, wheeling the garbage can back to its place in the garage next to a rack of mops, brooms, shovels, and rakes. He removes the plastic bag wrapped around the newspaper, putting it aside for later use by our neighbors, Joann and Mickey Chassey, to pick up the droppings of their Shih Tzu, Muffin.

Stephen presses the button to lower the garage door and enters the house again. He goes to the glass table in the breakfast nook and places the paper to the left side of his wife's plate and cereal bowl, which, to be helpful, he had set out the night before. At last Stephen goes to the kitchen to plug in the coffee maker and switch it on. Stephen had filled the coffee maker the night before, right after setting the breakfast table.

Stephen, my Dad, returns to the master bedroom to commence his hygiene, which my mother will help him complete.

The day is upon us.

PUBLISHER'S CLEARINGHOUSE

The red flag on the Keith's mailbox usually stood upright because Barbara mailed out an endless stream of payments and replies to Publisher's Clearinghouse. Whether the envelopes that Barbara sealed with special Publisher's Clearinghouse stickers all contained small checks made out to the publisher was none of my business. These pieces of correspondence preserved the illusion that someday a van full of people would arrive at the front door, ring the doorbell, and present the Keith family with balloons and a check for $10 million. Publisher's Clearinghouse had informed the Keiths that they were among the ten finalists in their region.

I did intervene at a certain point—when it became apparent that the mail-order companies were taking advantage of the indecisiveness of elderly people. I must have moved in with my parents during the heyday as the barrage of packages arrived, all containing items that no one had ordered. The problem was that Barbara paid for every item they sent her, faithfully mailing off a check. She purchased scissors, garden tools, an audio transmitter with headphones for the television (which I connected for her), even a hearing aid that she pinned to her shirt and connected to her ears with plastic buds and she wore until its point of failure.

At my suggestion, Barbara called Publisher's Clearinghouse to ask about the products that were being mailed to us, but the lady on the phone told Barbara that the mail order companies were independent and Publisher's Clearinghouse had nothing to do with it. I offered my mother and father another solution: to refuse the mail. I stacked the latest boxes by the mailbox with "refused" written on them in black marker.

And Barbara spoke to Mick, the mail carrier, telling Mick that she and her husband were old and didn't want all these things coming to their house. Mick, local hero to the Keith family, put an end to it, cutting off the flow of packages before they were ever delivered to Pineneedles Drive.

"Can you help me with something?" Barbara said.

She called me into the master bathroom. Sunlight poured through a semicircular window above an heirloom bureau. In the bathroom area around Barbara's lavatory—opposite Stephen's lavatory—the off-white wall and the white shag rug were splashed with red liquid.

"Don't ask me how I managed to do it," she said.

As red as freshly drawn blood, the streak of color had been shaken from a bottle of cosmetics. On the white background, the action of the red stains looked like the result of violence or impatience.

In a moment of paranoia, I thought that Barbara might be testing me.

This mess looked impossible. It looked unlikely. It looked like someone had created it deliberately.

I worked on the stains for quite a while, trying a variety of cleaning compounds. The key ingredient turned out to be beeswax that I rubbed into the shag, lifting the stains. I had found three jars of beeswax under the kitchen sink, all marked with the logo of Publisher's Clearinghouse.

I tried to be patient, but I found myself correcting my mother in a scolding fashion after she spilled maple syrup into the gap between the stove and the kitchen counter. Without a thorough cleaning, the syrup spill would attract ants. There was already a Silk Road for little black ants leading from the far end of the garage, up the wall near the light switch, through the seal of the door, and into the kitchen. We shouldn't provide the ants with any high-energy nutrition.

The cleanup was simple, the whole problem quite minor. I told Barbara, if she needed to decant syrup into a container, to be sure to do it over the sink in case it spilled. But I was uptight and I repeated my statement word for word, and that hurt her feelings because it was bossy.

I used the exact tone of voice that I had tried to avoid using, the voice of the stronger person upbraiding and attacking the weaker one.

I found out that Barbara had mixed Windex glass cleaner into the bottle of Dawn dish soap. While scrubbing some pots and pans in the kitchen sink, I saw little black delineations like crystalline structures floating in the bottle of liquid detergent. Sure enough, the smell and consistency of the dish soap had changed, altered by the glass cleaner.

Both substances were blue, and the blue jugs of each liquid that we purchased at Sam's Club stood side by side in the garage.

This bothered me because it spelled poison that all of us could absorb.

So I changed out the dish detergent, and I substituted golden-tinted Windex for the blue. I showed the gold liquid to Barbara, and told her, this time in a kindly manner, to use the gold stuff when she sprayed her glass table-tops.

I took the mixture of Windex and dish soap and used it to wash my car and to clean my golf clubs.

PERSISTENT
THOUGHTS

———— ··❖·· ————

S tephen Keith called Florida "a great place to live while you're starving to death." I've never heard a more apt description. Unless you are able to make a profit from selling property, Florida is not a thriving economic environment. I underestimated the difficulty of finding and keeping a job in Florida. Here, the "boss man" is everything and the worker nothing. People routinely work for minimum wage. People are transferred from one location to another far away all the time. Commuting within Florida is time-consuming and grueling. If you don't like it, you can quit because there's a line a mile long waiting to hold your job.

In fact, my move to Florida was more an emotional compulsion than a rational decision.

The weather was drenched and overcast the morning I packed my

Nissan 200SX. I drove north from Portland, Maine, to Brunswick to pick up Jim Bouchard, a friend who agreed to barrel down the eastern seaboard with me. So I began the trip driving thirty-two miles in the opposite direction.

By the time we hit Maryland that evening, we'd plunged into a giant rainstorm that stretched north all the way from Miami. At dusk, I tried to use the AC to clear the windshield, but the Nissan had lost its charge of Freon. In the lamplight-streaked dark, an SUV had to swerve to avoid rear-ending a disabled car, despite the glowing emergency markers that had been placed on the road, and nearly smashed into us. The motels in Baltimore were full, so we took a room at the Holiday Inn in Columbia, Maryland, and ended up drinking in the lounge in the midst of a wedding party.

The next morning, I was driving in a torrential downpour when the linkage to the windshield wipers came apart. I steered off the highway, Jim guiding me with his head out the passenger window. We wasted precious hours at a Pep Boys, watching Olympic soccer on TV. David Beckham bent in a goal for England. The linkage couldn't be fixed, but Jim balanced the gear together with a piece of plastic the size of a Jefferson nickel, and we drove south, the wipers moving constantly on the slow setting. Jim's wife, Alexandra, called him every couple hours giving us updates on the storm.

Having lost time in Maryland, by ten at night we only reached Dillon, South Carolina. On a lark, Jim wanted to stay at Pedro's South of the Border motel, and I pulled the Nissan off the highway and into a confusion of neon lights and souvenir shops. I parked, then I staggered to the motel lobby.

Crossing South Carolina and heading into Georgia the next morning, we burst out of the storm like superhuman babies out of an amniotic sac. The windows and sunroof let in a torrent of moist air warmed by sunshine. Jim's bald head was overpowered by the rays, so he wanted to stop to administer sunscreen.

Lifting the trunk hood, I dug between the suitcases and soft luggage topped with shirts still on their hangers. I had sold everything I owned except indispensable items: the framed art prints wrapped in newspaper, the guitar and guitar stand, a carry-on bag filled with ibuprofen, condoms, and sunscreen.

The warmth set us free to ramble. As Jim was driving I listened to his political rundowns and to the blues on Sirius radio. I let the pale shade of the pavement, the yellow grass, the green of the Georgia pines, and the delicate blue sky stream under my eyelids, sensing that my inner nature was an empty space more transient than the land around me, a space susceptible to insecurity and doubt, vulnerable to anxiety that had not materialized but waited in the wings.

I called Mom and Dad to let them know when I would arrive and that a friend was coming with me and that he would sleep overnight and go home the next day.

Stephen and Barbara Keith had slipped from one "plateau" of well-being to another several years back. The progression of Stephen's Parkinson's disease had brought their physical exercise to a screeching halt. They no longer walked the half-mile loop around the block, and Stephen began to resent Barbara playing golf with the ladies and leaving him by himself. They both had faded out of the realm of elderly, functioning people and slipped into a state of frailty. It was as if they had walked off a cliff but hadn't yet dropped through the air.

Stung by uncertainty as I debated moving to Florida to help them, I kept having the thought that I should "show some sympathy" to Stephen and Barbara. It was a persistent thought that cropped up during my martial arts practice. I had read Gavin deBecker and other writers on the subject of fear, so I paid attention to the nagging thought which deBecker related to the power of intuition.

In May of 2006 the City of Portland conducted an HIP, or heavy item pickup, and the streets of the city became lined with mattresses, appliances, and wooden furniture with the lamination separating.

The Munjoy Hill neighborhood where I lived, the site of a fiery betrayal and massacre of early colonists during the French and Indian Wars, was the first zone scheduled for HIP. I hauled a loveseat to the curb leaving it to languish in a steady drizzle. I abandoned a steamer trunk that I had used since I left home for college as a teenager. As the HIP shifted to other neighborhoods, I drove around town dumping things in various locations. I loaded my weight set into my car, drove to the correct zone, and left the weights on the sidewalk fully-assembled and ready for use. Boxes of books that had not sold in my yard sale were added to other people's rain-soaked piles.

I needed to reduce my personal inventory, and heavy things were the first to go. The coin collection my father had given me a number of years ago was heavy, but the burden seemed more metaphorical than material. The collection was housed in a cosmetics case which once belong to my maternal grandmother, Rena Moore. When he gave it to me, my father had assured me that there were "no strings attached," but I felt guilty after I sold it. I thought about the gold American dollar and the rare half-cents that Stephen Keith had accumulated. I felt like a palpable betrayer.

Stephen and Barbara Keith loved golf and football. During his high school years, Steve Keith played right tackle, and he also kicked off. He was the first player from Newport High School to make the State All-State team and was offered a full scholarship to play tackle at the University of Nevada. Steve never played for the Nevada Wolves, though. He chose instead to join the Navy as a member of the Silent Service in the War in the Pacific.

Although they had raised me as a New York Giants fan, Barb and Steve had rooted for twenty years now for the perennial underdog Tampa Bay Buccaneers. I knew they would be impressed with Jim, who was a placekicker for the semi-pro team, Midcoast Chaos.

Jim and I hit thunderstorms on I-75 on June 27, 2006, the day we arrived in Florida. On I-75, drivers tailgated one another in the morass of the downpour. We drove past eight rear-end collisions.

There was a wreck across the median, and a lady was trapped inside her vehicle. An ambulance had stopped, and EMTs were administering to the lady through the driver's side window. To complicate matters, a sixteen-wheel semi carrying a load of new cars had veered off the hardtop, its left tires sinking into wet sand, the cab of the semi flipping onto its side. One of the new cars had flown off the car carrier and now lay balanced on top of the ambulance. We saw the driver of the semi trapped inside his cab, but so far no one was helping him.

When I pulled the car into the Keiths' driveway, Stephen and Barbara were ready to greet us, standing just inside the open bay of the garage. They looked fine and healthy in their light Florida-appropriate apparel. Stephen wore his wrap-around anti-glaucoma sunglasses, and Barbara's hair was swept to one side in a casual style I had never seen on her. The hairstyle made her look youthful. As I got out of the car, the moment felt awkward. I felt as if I were forcing something into existence and making a huge error in judgment. My parents appeared to be two people who, at the time, didn't need any help. Later, I found out that Barbara had styled her hair that way as a quick fix only because she had missed her hair appointment.

I was grubby. I needed a shower. I carried many armfuls of stuff into the house, relieving the Nissan of its burden of tackle-boxes, firearms, printer and documents, and winter-style workout gear I would rarely wear while in Florida.

I showered, opened a beer. Barbara poured a screwdriver for Jim since Stephen's vision was bad, and he was clumsy at mixing drinks. Stephen took Jim into the master bedroom and showed him our family's military service medals mounted in a frame and, high on the wall above the sliding door to the master bath, the two framed photographs of the USS *Ray*, USS 271, my father's submarine, dramatically surfacing through whitecaps on a gray-scale ocean. After dinner, we watched a segment of a television miniseries, *Into the West*, a depiction of the hardships and brutalities of migration across the prairies. After that, Stephen and Barbara went to bed, Jim took a shower, and I capitulated in exhaustion and canceled our plans to drive to Ruby Tuesday's for another drink. We sat up for a while watching Canadian football.

The next morning I drove Jim to TPA to fly home. In the driveway, as Jim took in the breeze buffeting the canopy of the Queen palms reflected in the windshield of my Nissan, he said, "Now, I'm starting to feel sorry for you."

It was late June weather, warm, caressing and coddling.

Jim admitted he could not make the move I was making. He told me that if the need arose, he would not be able to help his own father. Several years ago, Jim's mother had died of cancer. His mother, Marge, had been a guiding light in Jim's life while his father had spoiled their relationship through insults and chronic negativity. Dropping Jim off at curbside at Jet Blue, it hit home that I had traded in a stable yet unsatisfying life for an uncertain present and an unknown future with my parents.

NEVERMORE

Eating breakfast together on Sunday mornings was part of family routine. Monday through Saturday, I brewed my coffee before Stephen and Barbara got up, and I'd head over to Starkey Park to exercise, letting them have their space together with Barbara reading Stephen the newspaper, both of them checking for action at the backyard bird feeder.

It was a heavy duty metal bird feeder, painted green, concealed against the foliage of the pine and candelabra trees nearby. If you didn't know it was there, you could turn and hit your head on it in broad daylight, as I did several times. One time, a Mexican worker smashed his head on it while driving a mower below the pine tree. In rage and frustration, he tore down the bird feeder and snapped the limb it was hanging from. I put it up again, though, hanging it from a nearby limb with a piece of chain.

I was taking a shower in the small bathroom that visitors used. Barbara was preparing breakfast—Sunday breakfast was a feast with bacon, eggs, melon, and Danish. I knew Stephen had taken his place at the table by the sound of packets of artificial sweetener being shaken and the toll of a teaspoon on the wall of his USS *Ray* coffee mug.

The shower in the small bathroom was funky. It had a nozzle that didn't generate much pressure and a door that rumbled when someone slid it open or closed.

I sat down at the table. I was not trying to scrutinize my father, but Stephen shook so much pepper onto his poached egg that it turned black. He couldn't taste food well due to his Parkinson's, so it didn't matter much. When he was done with the salt and pepper, he looked at me and my mother.

"I heard a sliding noise up on the roof," he said, gesturing. "I thought it was Chris."

It was odd that Stephen had not recognized the rumble of the shower door in the small bathroom, having lived in the house for fourteen years at that point. It seemed strange that my father would believe that the source of the sliding noise was me climbing on the roof of the house and making repairs before the neighborhood was stirring. It was a key to how he perceived me, a clue given in a Freudian slip: his son scrambling overhead, crawling all over the place, "taking over," or at least attempting to.

A little path like a deer trail ran through the St. Augustine turf between the Keiths' house and the Stams' next door. In steamy sunshine all morning and in moist shade in the afternoon, the groove of the trail resulted in part from Stephen's many journeys to the backyard to clean the birdbath and to refill the bird feeder. The task brought into use a rickety stepladder stained with white paint and a dull green, plastic bowl with a spout, filled with black oil sunflower seeds.

Like other elements of Stephen's routine, the task was a practical part of maintaining the home, an important contribution. Wearing his dark, protective sunglasses, khaki shorts, polo shirt and moccasins, Stephen filled the bird feeder, retrieved the mail, administered weed killer to the lawn, sprayed poison into ant hills in the sidewalk cracks, and watered the flower beds and hedges. Once in a while he used the power washer to clean the outside windows. He usually experienced a burst of energy after taking his Parkinson's medication in the morning and got something done before settling into his recliner in front of the television set.

One day while Stephen was getting ready to fill the bird feeder and was making his way along the little path between the houses, a crow had alighted on the Stams' roof and had perched there. It had spoken to him just like a person carrying on a conversation, so he said.

When I heard the story of the crow, I pressed my father to tell me what the crow had said, or what he thought it had said. Stephen only smiled and didn't answer me.

I was intrigued. This story, this visitation, felt like some kind of breakthrough. The phrase that came to mind was, of course, Poe's "Nevermore," in "The Raven", suggestive as it was of a disintegrating mental state. Could a messenger "from the Night's Plutonian shore" have arrived at Pineneedles Drive in broad daylight? I wondered.

I was reminded of my father reciting "Quoth the Raven, 'Nevermore'" to me and my siblings when we were children and reciting stanzas from other poems exploring solitude and survival, "The Wreck of the Piccadilly

Daisy" and "The Rime of the Ancient Mariner".

Month after month, Barbara had watched her husband through the arched window by the glass table, worried when Stephen climbed the shaky stepladder to fill the bird feeder. One day she told me that Stephen had tripped and fallen in the grass and that I was to take over the task of refilling the bird feeder.

A WWII submarine vet and former football player, a man who with great effort had supported his wife and five children, Stephen could no longer negotiate the thick turf of the yard.

In 1988, the man who had run aground in a submarine on Honshu, the Japanese mainland, who had worked for twenty years as a State Police office and wrestled drunks to the ground, migrated south from Vermont driving a rented truck and towing a car. Their eldest son and their eldest daughter, Stephen and Alison, followed them in Stephen's, the son's, Volkswagen Jetta, keeping in touch with the Keiths by walkie-talkie.

Retirement wasn't Stephen's first choice. Before retiring, he had applied for a transfer to Miami but didn't get the job—as a member of a U.S. Customs Service SWAT team whose mission was to board ships suspected of carrying narcotics.

A mood of regret tainted the first phase of his retirement.

Initially, Barbara was appalled by the ramshackle garages and tattoo parlors lining U.S. Route 19 in Hudson and Port Richey, but she soon got used to Florida. She loved the balmy night air of southern climes, anyway, having traveled to Submarine Veterans reunions in Mobile and having gambled in Biloxi. Her son Stephen owned a house in Key West. Alison, in no hurry to return north, rented an apartment near the Keiths and lived there for four years.

The Keiths moved from house to house, as they always had done. Country Club Drive in Hudson was their first home in the Sunshine State, a tidy, landscaped property in a quiet neighborhood by appearance. The yellowing grass and vehicles parked on the lawns really did not denote that street fights would erupt directly in front of the house at night—a jeans jacket flailing against an Arkansas toothpick. And there was no way to know except by anecdotal evidence—and they hadn't spoken to any of the neighbors—that on a frosty night in winter they would hear footsteps crunching past the bedroom windows and a hand trying the doorknobs of the kitchen and side doors.

Not long after the Keiths had moved to Florida, their son, Stephen, my older brother, committed suicide. The subject of a police investigation at Springfield College in Massachusetts, without alerting anyone in the family to the crisis, Stephen drank several bottles of fine wine, sealed his garage door airtight with duct tape, got into the Mazda MX6 parked inside the garage, settled into the driver's seat with a can of Diet Pepsi, turned the ignition, let the engine of the car run, and asphyxiated himself.

Barbara was devastated by her son's death. Stephen had been a kind, intelligent person, an electrician who designed and installed AC systems. He had a successful life as the head of the physical plant at Springfield College.

I was stunned. Following my brother's suicide, I plunged into a state of all-encompassing negativity. I saw human endeavor as hopeless and trivial in the face of death and decay. I was kept going only by the strength of routine of my karate practice. Daily life had become a permanent, Buddhist contemplation of the skeleton, anticipating the work of time.

Right after it happened, some mornings I woke up feeling refreshed and cleansed, and for a split second I felt at ease, then with sudden power the weight of my brother's death fell upon me again and I felt ashamed that I had forgotten that my brother was dead, forgotten that our family's good fortune had been shattered.

With proceeds from my brother's life insurance policy, my parents were able to get away from the street fights in Hudson. They bought a home on Ironwood Circle in Bayonet Point, paying cash for the property, cash that Barbara decried as "blood money."

It was a three-bedroom home with a full-sized pool under a lanai. The backyard, bordered by a creek and given shape by bushes and trees, merged with the rough of the eighth hole at Beacon Woods Golf Course.

Membership at Beacon Woods Golf Course was prohibitively expensive, though, so Stephen purchased a family membership at a tiny, hardscrabble course nearby, also called Ironwood, where he and Barbara played, along with his brothers, my uncles Dick and Clyde, joined on occasion by my sister, Alison.

While living on Ironwood Circle, Barbara's knees deteriorated, and she underwent the replacement that would keep her on her feet for eighteen more years, playing golf for fifteen of them. To her credit, Barbara pursued an aggressive therapy regimen, doubling the normal number of repetitions she performed in her swimming pool.

She told me she had made the right decision getting both knees replaced at once. The pain had been so fierce that she never would have gone back to do the other one.

The size of the house and the upkeep of the pool factored into the Keiths' decision to move again. In 1992 Alison found a choice pleasant model home for them on a double lot on Pineneedles Drive in River Ridge.

Their lives had entailed a half-marathon of moves—by the time I graduated high school in Beaconsfield, Quebec, in 1969, I had attended six schools and had lived in eleven houses.

The Keiths' former residences all had been in Vermont, Quebec, and Florida, and their final move to Pineneedles Drive marked the twenty-third notch in the family belt.

CARD GAMES

———— ·❖· ————

After moving to Pineneedles Drive, Stephen and Barbara experienced a social resurgence. They hosted card parties with their neighbors, the Chasseys, the Dolans and the Golattas. The social calendar fell into place with ease. Couples came over for drinks on very little advance notice. Billy and Edna Williams visited from Jacksonville, Billy being Stephen's shipmate aboard the USS *Ray*. They drove to Sarasota to visit Uncle Bud and Aunt Tess Nealy. Once in a while, Jonesy, Stephen's old friend from his tenure with the Vermont State Police, and Jonesy's wife, Charlene, showed up bearing Charlene's homemade bread and crafts that she had fashioned out of plaster and artificial flowers.

Events rolled along as the pages of the calendar turned. Barbara and Jeanne, Dick's wife and a friend of Barbara's since childhood, joined a flower arranging club, but they quit following their first high-pressure annual flower show. Barbara's moth orchid garnered an orange ribbon, one of three given out for Best of Show.

They took out mortgages on their home to buy cars and to fly to Aruba with their neighbors Peggy and Jack Dolan and Mickey and Joann Chassey, who lived right across the street. The Chasseys were younger than the Keiths. Mickey had served in the Navy, too, but he hadn't engaged in any combat operations, an important distinction among servicemen. In Aruba, they watched young couples dance and got out on the dance floor themselves and held each other as in days of old. Stephen got inebriated and made fun of Barbara for her speaking so admiringly of the "trade winds."

In their hearts they were nowhere close to needing one of their children to join them. They walked the half mile loop in Tall Pines each morning, deeded their home to their four children, drove to their doctor's appointments, played golf and planned more trips to Biloxi and Aruba.

One night they held a card party. Vinnie and Maddy Golatta had come over, along with the Chasseys and the Dolans. The Golattas were a wonderful couple, with Maddy six feet tall, thin as a wisp. With her white hair and her royal bearing, she towered over Vinnie, a short solid Italian with a black mustache. It was a card game on a timeless fall evening. The humidity was low, so the doors were left open and the laughter of the players floated on the night air.

Before long, though, Maddy experienced chest pains. She took her nitroglycerine. Then she became pale and clammy, and her pulse dropped. Joann Chassey, a nurse, called 911, and an ambulance and a fire truck rushed to Pineneedles Drive to attend to Maddy.

Stephen said, "When the Keiths have a party, you can expect to see a rescue wagon."

But within a few months Maddy's physical and mental health deteriorated. She was placed in a ward where she stayed in her bed and recognized none of her visitors, including Vinnie.

Then followed a cascade of losses. Jack Dolan died from complications of diabetes. Peggy Dolan, a good friend of Barbara's, lived in the neighborhood for a while longer. Peggy's daughter, Patty, an aerobics instructor in Georgia, was an alcoholic. She tried to sober up, but she fell in love with another alcoholic and lost custody of her own daughter. Peggy secluded herself in her home up the block, letting unopened mail and unread newspapers accumulate in piles on her living room floor. Eventually, her relatives moved Peggy into an assisted living facility in Clearwater. News of Peggy trickled in from time to time, but Barbara never saw Peggy again.

Jeanne Keith, my aunt and Barbara's best friend, died from an aneurysm in 1998. A year later, her husband, Dick, passed away. Stephen and Barbara traveled north for both of those funerals

When they visited Ludlow, Vermont, in 1999, Barbara stated that she was now in her "dotage," citing her memory loss, and Stephen seemed frail and his gait halting.

Over the years, Stephen had functioned with one good eye and one eye that had been damaged, he claimed, in his boyhood when he had stared at a solar eclipse. This left him with a blind spot, like tunnel vision in reverse, in his right eye.

Following a trip to Aruba, Stephen underwent a cornea transplant that left him with a herpes Zoster infection in his eye. In his good eye. The pressure in his eye skyrocketed damaging his retina, leaving him blind.

As a result, Barbara took over the driving.

As if that were not enough, he could no longer walk a hundred yards without pain. His shortened steps became a shuffle. Getting out of the passenger side of the car, he dragged the rubber soles of his moccasins across the parking lot outside Publix supermarket. Once a physically powerful man, Stephen was now diagnosed with Parkinson's disease.

With his low vision, he had relied on golfing partners to help him align his shots. Now, with the onset of muscular stiffness due to Parkinson's, he couldn't make solid contact, couldn't put the club face on the ball.

My father introduced me to the game of golf when I was a kid. We used to play nine holes at a time at Newport Country Club just before sunset when the course was empty. I remember sitting on the living room floor as my parents pointed out the idiosyncrasies of Chi Chi Rodriguez, the ever-black apparel of Gary Player, the Army that trailed Arnold Palmer, and we rooted for Palmer as he endured the onslaught of that brash newcomer, Jack Nicklaus.

At Christmas in 2003 I begged my father to play nine holes with me. He reluctantly agreed to go out. We went to River Ridge, the little course nearby where Barbara and Stephen used to play three times a week. I clung to nostalgia for a few holes until I realized that Stephen could not strike the ball and wasn't enjoying himself.

The half-mile walk they took each morning fell by the wayside. Barbara drove to all their appointments, and she gave up her own golf game in fear of making her husband jealous. With the adverse personality changes that came with middle-stage Parkinson's, Stephen resented any time that Barbara spent without him. Without the morning walks and the physical activity of golf, Barbara was getting weaker, too.

They lost more family members, Barbara's brother, Charles Moore, in 1994, Charles' wife, Delores, in 2001, Stephen's brother, Clyde, in 2004.

They grew lonely and frightened. Thinking that my sister, Andrea, and I were trying to take their house away from them, Stephen and Barbara insisted that we deed the house back to them. So we did.

Fewer people visited. The Chasseys didn't come over for drinks any more. Instead, they sought the company of new arrivals to the Tall Pines subdivision, people who were younger and healthier than the Keiths. The Keiths kept to their routine. Barbara read the newspaper to Stephen each morning at the breakfast table. Unless physical discomfort paralyzed him, Stephen performed chores around the yard or went grocery-shopping with Barbara. By late morning, Stephen sought the stability of his recliner and turned on the television set and blasted the volume.

The days of painting directional arrows on the slab of concrete in the back yard and cementing Canadian quarters to the garage floor were over. Even in the first year or two of his diminished eyesight, Stephen could be found buffing his white Cadillac to a soft polish in the shade of the garage. Now he never went near the car. Barbara drove their 2003 Mercury Sable, and the chamois cloths languished in a dusty paper bag on a shelf above the sack of sunflower seeds.

Barbara plotted what needed to be done. She kept up with housework and cooking. She rested for hours in her recliner, working on word puzzles to take her mind off her stress.

They felt that they needed to move again. Barbara kept a folder of pamphlets and fliers from assisted living facilities tucked next to her basketful of word puzzles. The Keiths sensed the end of their residency in Tall Pines. They didn't know where to go. There were uncertainties but one thing was sure: bonded by mutual love or some other form of emotional entanglement, they had each other.

EYE DROPS

---◆---

One morning while Barbara was working on word puzzles, I called her into my bedroom. She came in and sat on the edge of the bed as I showed her some pictures I had taken in the wilderness park, quasi-dramatic shots of cypress knees soaking in the Cotee River where it was only a strand.

I glanced through the bedroom doorway. Just out of sight, Stephen stood listening to us, not aware that he was fully reflected in a hallway mirror that hung outside the little bathroom. He wanted to find out if we were talking about him. He realized that he had undergone dramatic changes—nerves in his brain were dying. His sense of balance had been destroyed. He was seeing things not actually there, remembering things that had not happened.

Barbara was hard of hearing. She had purchased hearing aids, shopping for them by herself, yet all the ones that she bought had failed. The latest failure had cost $500. Stephen didn't want her to buy any more hearing aids. To help Barbara hear the television, he played it at top volume, which undoubtedly resulted in more hearing loss to both of them.

As part of family routine, I joined my parents after supper to watch *Everybody Loves Raymond* followed by *Jeopardy*. Years ago, they had worn out their interest in *Seinfeld* in like manner, watching the same show night after night. I was teaching evening or "night" classes as well as day classes, so it was fun to sit around with Stephen and Barbara. Later Stephen called me in from my bedroom to watch boxing and UFC. I was glad we did something together, even if it was watching television. I twisted and stuffed bright yellow foam earplugs into my ears for protection.

Barbara showed me books on Parkinson's disease, and I read them. She kept the books hidden in a sewing basket under a chair in my bedroom. She didn't want Stephen to read them. She didn't want him to find out about the cruel prognosis in the later stages of Parkinson's, how he risked degenerating to a state of bedridden, incontinent helplessness. In bed each night, she read Stephen a chapter from a book, often on the topic of submarines. When I first moved in with them, Barbara was reading him *The Terrible Hours*, the story of Swede Momsen developing the "Momsen Lung" which had been used in 1939 to rescue sailors from the USS *Squalus* off the coast of New Hampshire.

Stephen needed eye drops to control intraocular pressure and the herpes Zoster infection. His eye drop regimen consisted of two drops in the morning and four drops at night, but two of the drops needed to be administered half an hour apart, and he couldn't do it by himself. The task of placing the drops into the correct eye, monitoring the supply, and refilling the prescriptions fell to Barbara, who referred to her handwritten list to keep her on track.

It was like running an outpatient clinic. Each morning, Stephen needed drops of brimonidine tartrate to help the eye to drain and timolol maleate to combat glaucoma. At night, Barbara administered the same drugs, along with drops of dexamethasone/tobramycine, a steroid and antibiotic, and latanoprost, another glaucoma battler.

Barbara ordered most of the medications from the VA and received them by mail in softly rattling bundles.

Barbara procured the carbidopa-levadopa for Stephen's idiopathic parkinsonism, atenol and Lisinopril for his hypertension, acyclovir tablets for the eye infection, and simvastatin to lower his cholesterol. She sorted the pills into green custard cups ahead of time and placed the pills on the table at mealtime.

With Barbara's permission I scoured the medicine cabinets and threw away bottles of cough syrup and pain relievers that had long expired.

Barbara was eighty, but she drove down U.S. 19 to St. Luke's Eye Clinic in Tarpon Springs with me in the passenger seat. Due to Barbara's low hearing, I spoke with the intake assistant at St. Luke's through a hole in the layer of glass. The assistant and I were both surprised to find that Barbara was attending her second appointment within the week.

We sat in an impeccably clean waiting area bordered with polished wooden handrails which helped the elderly patients get around. We looked at large oil paintings of the Anclote wetlands whose pewter and green grasses were themselves visible below the office windows. Barbara thought she heard herself being called and stood up a few times before her turn came.

As with the other patients, it took over an hour for Barbara to be seen by the screening nurse. Then she came back and sat for another half hour. At last a kindly-spoken mid-tier ophthalmologist took her to an examining room.

Shelves full of new copies of Dr. Gill's motivational books were available free to all who wanted them. Dr. Gill was a writer and a marathon runner. The medical clinic was founded upon Gill's spirituality. A Christian undercurrent ran through the business to the extent that prayer meetings were held with the staff before each shift, and the support staff gave earnest testimony on television of how Dr. Gill had helped them come to grips with the pain of living and to straighten out their lives.

I felt full of purpose and optimism in support of my mother. I met a middle-aged woman from Georgia who had brought her substantially older husband to the Clinic. While Barbara and the woman's husband were both being attended to, the woman and I drank coffee and conversed. The St. Luke's staff brought out muffins still warm from the oven.

She was a raven-haired, fair skinned beauty wearing, though it was July, a tight-fitting turtleneck sweater, the type of sweater that is not even for sale in Florida. From her fresh, expertly-applied makeup and her diamond ring and other jewelry, I could tell she was a woman of means. We exchanged stories of what had brought us to the Clinic. She was the first person I had met in Florida, and I thought that meeting her might be a sign of better things to come—in my social life, that is. But that didn't turn out to be the case.

The doctor had given Barbara eye drops in order to dilate her pupils, so I drove us home. Barbara had been driving on the Sun Coast of

Florida for years. Ironically, U.S. Route 19 is one of deadliest highways in the United States because of the cut-throughs across three lanes of traffic to enable motorists to get to the crumbling, stucco-faced pawn shops, the car dealerships, the tattoo parlors, and the Mrs. Mobility motorized wheelchair store. All the elderly drivers mix poorly with the throng of high school students driving up and down U.S. 19 and the tractor trailers running through intersections at 60 mph as the traffic signals change. U.S. 19 is a stew of local traffic—Lexuses, classic Ferrari kits, muscle cars, cars with dented panels and loud exhausts, even dune buggies with handwritten, "tag stolen," license plates.

Barbara donned protective sunglasses and offered me a pair of disposable sunglasses that were in the glove compartment of the car.

"It's hard having someone stay in the house with us," she said.

"We don't get along very well," I said.

"Let me tell you when I need help," she said, "and just relax about it the rest of the time."

Barbara suggesting that I stay in the passing lane on Ridge Road for miles because we needed to be in that lane to make our turn.

"Daddy's not himself. At times, it's like living with a different person. You can see it, can't you? That's not him. He's jealous of you playing golf. He's jealous of you spending any time at all with me."

I tried to imagine what Stephen was going through. From what I had read in Barbara's books, clumps of protein were forming in his brain resulting in loss of nerve function. One could see the stiffness in his physical movement. His face was a stony mask of displeasure.

"A lady that lives around the corner had to put her husband in a home. He had Parkinson's. He got mad at everything she did," Barbara said, "and he beat her up."

I put the disposable sunglasses Barbara had given me into a drawer in my bedroom.

Later, Barbara retrieved a book of old family photographs that I had never looked at. It was a thin volume bound with cord, the pictures matted with black construction paper. Parents, children, cousins, people who had lived long before me posed in the richly toned photographs. Barbara told me about some of them. They were people of my own blood line, predecessors who had lived honest lives, suffered emotions, visited places now lost or transformed, engaged in events so numerous and intricate it seemed like Barbara was narrating a tide of history that I could not encapsulate.

She showed me a picture of three of Stephen's great-aunts at a long-forgotten outing on Seymour Lake in Morgan, Vermont. It was a moody image of three women wearing fur coats and hats, attractive yet unsmiling women leaning elbow-to-elbow against a boulder on the beach, the pine woods and water behind them giving way to the shadows of a late summer evening.

PAIN PILLS

---·◈·---

Amid a cluster of pill vials on the sunlit white kitchen counter, beside green custard cups containing allotments of Parkinson's medications, sat Barbara's amber-colored vial of hydrocodone. This was the cache from which her handy bedside supply was replenished. Hydrocodone supplemented the Oxycontin she had been prescribed to control headaches caused by the giant cell arteritis which was a side effect related to her polymyalgia rheumatica, or PMR. The headaches were fierce. Barbara likened them to having nails driven through her eyes.

Barbara split the hydrocodone tablets in half using her blue pill cutter and filled a heart-shaped china container with the pill segments. She kept the heart-shaped container on her bed stand, and she usually took a half tablet after getting into bed at night to help her fall asleep.

Barbara's prescriptions, apart from the ones she kept track of for

Stephen, included meclizine for dizziness, nortriptylin to calm her and help her sleep, Prednisone to reduce the pain of arthritis, ventolin to fuel her nebulizer, Nexium for acid indigestion, Benicar for high blood pressure, and Diltiazem CD to control heart rhythm. She also possessed an Advair inhaler.

And she routinely filled the dermatologist Dr. Natalie Lama Monticciolo's prescriptions for anti-bacterial agents: Biafine, cephalexin, gentamicin, azithromycin and Mupirocin.

In addition, Stephen and Barbara daily consumed low dose Bayer aspirin—intended to thin their blood—aspirin which would factor into Stephen's undoing.

Part of my role, as I misconstrued it, was to convince my parents to take fewer medications. I thought that taking pain killers on top of the other medications might be contributing to my mother's mental confusion.

When I suggested that she reconsider all the medications she was taking, Barbara countered by describing her piercing, giant cell headaches.

"We love you, Chris, but you're not a doctor," she said.

"He's not a doctor," Stephen said, "even if he does play one on television."

In recent years I'd noticed my parents indulging in a sort of baby talk, a willful abandonment of the specific words for specific things. Avid birdwatchers, they now referred to goldfinches merely as "yellow birds." Barbara used the word "thing" over and over again.

Barbara was having trouble remembering her vocabulary, and it happened often. When Mary Keith, my Uncle Clyde's fifth wife, came over for dinner, I sensed Barbara's embarrassment as she waived her turn in dinner conversation, stuck on a word. Sometimes I filled in her words for her, even in the presence of company, knowing exactly what my mother was trying to say, knowing what direction she was going in.

One day after lunch, while preparing a grocery list and speaking aloud each item before she wrote it down, Barbara hesitated on a word with a sibilant first consonant, saying "ssssss . . . ," and the syllable wavered and lasted until it became suspenseful as to what she would pronounce, and I was leaning toward her as if to help push the word through her larynx, which word turned out to be "cereal." I observed this with alarm.

A few nights after I had first arrived in Florida, a few nights after I had cleaned the red nail polish off a white wall and from a white shag carpet, I sat on the couch watching television with Stephen. Barbara stood at the white kitchen counter laying out her hydrocodone tablets and counting them and marking the days on a calendar to see how many tablets she was supposed to have. Over two dozen of her hydrocodone tablets were missing, and she asked me if I had taken them.

"I have to ask," she said.

"I'm not in the habit of taking other people's prescription medications," I retorted. "I'm not David."

I regretted the words as soon as I had spoken them. David was my cousin, Clyde's son. David was close to me in age, and he and his older brother, Kit, were blood brothers to me as kids.

As the children in my generation grew up, many of us used alcohol or took drugs, sometimes excessively. The same was true of David.

David had earned his living as a kitchen supply and cutlery salesman. He was a genuinely sweet person, a favorite of my mother and father. He had lived in Jacksonville with his wife, Ruth Ann, who worked at the Jacksonville Jaguars. At least, they lived there until Ruth Ann started taking out-of-town trips with her boss and began cheating on David.

After his divorce, David's drinking increased, and for long periods of time he moved about from crash pads to seedy motels in Florida. He failed in his efforts to remain clean.

At one point he got a job as a dock worker at a marina. There was an accident one day when a yacht owned by Jack Nicklaus pulled into the marina and tried to moor. David was trapped against the dock, and he injured his knee. He collected quite a bit of money in a legal settlement. He quit the job and moved aimlessly from place to place. He didn't get in touch with anyone in the family for a long time.

After Uncle Clyde's death in 2004, however, the family had hired detectives to locate David. Detectives found David in a motel room in Fort Lauderdale, dead from a heroin overdose. Clyde and David, father and son, were buried side by side on a summer day in Newport, Vermont. I spoke on behalf of David at the funeral.

There was no justification, except the root of my own selfishness and insecurity, for my saying something hurtful to the memory of my cousin who had died only two years ago. Yet my self-doubt was so great, my emotions so raw, that I lashed out knowing that my mother and father had loved David. And as a child, I had loved him, too.

As for the hydrocodone, it turned out that Barbara had miscalculated and none were missing.

MODERN TIMES

—◆—

I drove Stephen to the Circle G Ranch on Plathe Road to buy black oil sunflower seeds. Massive sacks of pungent grain lined the walls and filled the loft overhead. Customers in boots and cowboy hats settled their accounts, and Stephen placed his order for a twenty-pound bag of seeds, fingering the bills in his wallet and collecting the change. I carried the bag to my Nissan, loaded it in the trunk, and steered up Little Road toward Decubellis, stopping at a 7-Eleven store on the way back so Stephen could buy lottery tickets.

Stephen pointed to a swamp along Decubellis Road. There was a large lovely pond circled with bulrushes and covered with water lilies.

"I have a recurring dream about that pond," he said. "A nightmare."

"What happens?" I said.

"I go out in a canoe and tip over and flounder," he said. "Then alligators close in on me."

When I pulled the car into the driveway, the remote control for the garage door wasn't working. The battery had lost its charge.

The Keiths kept their front door locked and bolted, always entering through the garage. Barbara was out driving somewhere, so she wasn't there to open the door.

"How do you get in the house," I asked, "if you get home and the power is out?"

"You don't!" Stephen exclaimed.

I considered this an unnecessary liability. I didn't want to get home in an electrical storm, tired or hungry or needing to defecate, and be stuck outside until the power was restored.

I took the battery out of the remote and shook it back and forth. I put in back in the remote and the door came up. I talked Stephen into leaving the front door unbolted during the day, so we could use the keys to enter through the front door if we had to.

I felt guilty about malingering on the golf course while the working folk of Florida toiled at their jobs, so until I started teaching I put everything I had into doing yard work for Stephen and Barbara.

I replaced log edger around Barbara's flower gardens. I pruned blighted sections of hedge and chopped suckers at the base of the white bird-of-paradise. I cleaned the gutters. I swept the garage, chasing little frogs from the piles of grass clippings in the corners.

I cleared the lower branches of our red maple using a reverse pull hand saw that Barbara had purchased from Publisher's Clearinghouse. I remember Barbara lifting the folding hand saw from the box and showing it to me.

"Is this something you could use?" she said.

I knew that I should send the saw back or pay for it myself.

"Yes," I said. "It's a beauty."

Then Barbara wrote out the check for $24.95.

To no avail, I suggested we remove the overgrown Yucca trees which were crowding our long leaf pines. We needed the canopies of the pines elevated; their branches extended too close to the roof now. We needed more tree work done.

In August I started teaching composition classes at Pasco-Hernando Community College. My classes were held at the tidy West Campus landscaped with azalea hedge and camellia bushes, with redbud, water oak and sycamore trees, the campus grounds dotted with karst limestone boulders. I liked reading and pronouncing the surnames of the students: Soto, Stokes, Stackhouse, Gozo and Santiago, names I had never used before, unlike the names of students in Maine and Vermont I had had whose surnames were Brochu, Pateneau, Parenteau, Pomerleau.

I ordered a copy of Bob Dylan's CD, *Modern Times*. When the mail carrier brought the package to our front door, I tore it open and held it up so Stephen and Barbara could see the cover art: daubs of city lights and a long white sedan rendered in a smear of time-exposure. I waved it in front of them.

I said, "This is a world-changing album!"

"Not for us," they said in unison.

I admired their steadfastness—their open defiance of contemporary nuance, their lack of outrage in the face of modern bluster and fraud.

It was the arc of their own lives that preoccupied them. Stephen had an aneurysm in his chest. Part of the family narrative had been that Stephen would drop dead on the golf course: at least he would die doing something he loved. But he didn't play golf any more.

The pressures of running the household exhausted Barbara. She made the doctor's appointments and drove to them, and the number of appointments was burgeoning. Stephen, too, went to St. Luke's Eye Clinic, and he had appointments at the VA eye clinic, at a heart specialist twice a year although nothing was wrong with his heart, at two separate doctors for his Parkinson's disease, at a podiatrist's office to have his toenails clipped. He also visited a retinal specialist at the VA.

These appointments were in addition to ones they had with their regular doctors. Besides the physical entrapment of keeping the appointments, the everyday presence of their ailments proved confounding. I had written down a phone number on a piece of scrap paper, and as I turned the paper over, I saw this note written in my mother's handwriting:

aneurysm

ulcer

intestines infection

swallowing

5 weeks

go to Publix pharmacy

The privilege of hearing about all Barbara's personal problems belonged to my sisters, but over time I became aware of most of her problems.

She had problems swallowing, like her husband whose chewing and swallowing problems were linked to parkinsonism. The tissue of her esophagus was rigid, and the muscles of her diaphragm were weak. As a result, her body couldn't pull food all the way down into her stomach. She had a procedure done at Morton Plant Northbay Hospital in New Port Richey. The gastroenterologist, Dr. Rodriguez, injected Botox along

Barbara's esophagus to soften the tissue. I drove her to Northbay and took her home afterward.

Dr. Rodriguez was a hero to Barbara. She had a letter from his office which was of great importance to her. It was a standard letter that all patients receive before they undergo a procedure, but this letter often surfaced next to Barbara's chair, on her bureau, on the counter next to the vials of pills. And from time to time she asked of the whereabouts of that letter.

The year before I moved to Florida, Barbara had suffered diarrhea for six months nonstop. My sister, Alison, and I got her to start taking GSE, grapefruit seed extract, that helped to control her diarrhea. Later she started buying lactate over the counter, but it was unclear whether a doctor ever diagnosed her lactose intolerance.

I helped Barbara balance the checkbook one time, but family finances were a taboo subject, a subject Stephen did not want me privy to, and I was not allowed to do it again.

Forgetfulness plagued Barbara. I was tricked more than once into arriving at a doctor's office with Barbara on the wrong day. At last I learned to call ahead to verify what she had written down in the squares on the calendar.

Maybe the novelty of my good will had worn off. Stephen decided he would not go to the grocery store with Barbara if I went along, saying Barbara did not need both of us with her. I wanted him to come with us to get him out of his chair. I felt like I was gypping him out of his chance to move his body and feel useful.

Stephen didn't want to ride to Homosassa Springs to look at alligators. He refused to ride over to Starkey Park to look at trees.

He exploded one morning when he saw me pouring orange juice, telling me it was his job. Not long after that, Stephen gave up that job for good because he couldn't see well enough to pour. He tried to pour juice into glasses which were turned upside down, their rims on the counter.

The arc of their lives was veering toward death, and death became part of their vocabulary.

When the lawn care crew had nearly denuded her split-leaf philodendron and cut back her bird-of-paradise, Barbara threw up her hands saying, "I might as well die."

Tall Pines sponsored a big yard sale, and Barbara sold lots of clothes. After sitting at their table in the garage all day, she and Stephen were tired out. Barbara told me, "That's the last time we're ever having a yard sale."

She said the same thing as the two of them toiled over a batch of chocolate fudge, Barbara wearing her apron and eyeglasses, confused over the ingredients, Stephen stirring mechanically.

"This is the last time we're ever making fudge," she said.

Although spoken in exasperation, it was an accurate prediction. Just as they had stated that the trip to Bow Lake, New Hampshire, was their "last vacation," they had assessed everything correctly. That was their final vacation, their final yard sale, their last batch of fudge.

I was in the garage cleaning golf clubs one afternoon when Barbara came out and rested her head on my shoulder, crying.

"I'd like to retire from life," she said, "but I don't know how."

I assured her that her daughters were working on finding a place for her—the project to put them in an assisted living cottage in Connecticut, though, would not pan out. That arrangement was prohibitively expensive.

We considered various scenarios. Stephen liked the idea of buying a villa, a smaller place, but Barbara knew she could not keep up with cooking and taking care of her husband and me, "the two of them," as she put it. It was taking Stephen longer and longer to complete his morning hygiene. He couldn't dress himself without help from Barbara.

My siblings and I had never thought through the process of what to do with our parents, or when to do it. We had not investigated the depth of their financial reserve or what my father's government health plan would cover.

Stephen didn't want to move, anyway. He had grown old and blind in his pleasant house. He knew where his bottles of pesticides lay in waiting, where the hoses hung in the garage, where dozens of extra flashlight batteries weighed down the shelves near the laundry room.

My goal was to keep my mother and father living in their own home as long as practicable. They were past the point of going into assisted living, beyond the stage of being able to learn a new routine. Stephen would be lost, and Barbara would be unable to figure out the appliances. When the time came, the next step for them was a nursing home.

During football season I played golf Sunday afternoons, leaving Stephen and Barbara to root for the Buccaneers in the comfort of their living room, Dad having his VO and Mom refilling the pretzel dish, cutting cheese, getting geared up for the fast food run that followed the game every Sunday.

Once the college bowl season rolled around, though, Stephen and I watched games together, including the January 2007 NCAA Championship between Ohio State and Florida.

He pulled up a chair about three feet from the television screen. The game came on, and Ohio State's Herb Ginn Jr. returned the opening kickoff for a touchdown, dealing Florida a telling blow on the first play of the game. Stephen sipped his VO and settled into his chair, and I wiggled into position on the couch, hoping for a Gator comeback. We had absorbed the worst possible opening. We were worried, but we took it without complaint.

Some fans felt that Florida hadn't qualified for the national championship game and that Michigan should have been playing.

Ohio State's roster was loaded with talent, including QB Troy Smith who won the Heisman Trophy that year.

Chris Leak was the starting quarterback for Florida, but on short yardage plays, the Gators brought in another quarterback, freshman Tim Tebow. Tebow contributed by throwing a one-yard touchdown pass and rushing for a one-yard touchdown. In the end, the Gators had beaten the Buckeyes 41-14.

The opposite of not seeing things well is to see things that are not there. Rising from his chair one night, Stephen walked toward the breakfast area where his award for making a hole-in-one on the eighth hole at River Ridge Golf Club hung on the white wall in the shadow. He seemed to be pointing at an area beneath the glass table.

"What do you see, Steve?" my mother asked. "A gecko?"

The Parkinson's sufferer may hallucinate small creatures darting about—when this happened Barbara would engage Stephen in conversation, asking him about what he was seeing, as her books had said she must do.

Another development in mid-stage Parkinson's is that the dream-world of the sufferer becomes indistinguishable from reality, as real if not more real than waking life.

When Stephen's old friend, Jonesy, and his wife, Charlotte, visited, Stephen told stories of their days together in the Vermont State Police, stories that Jonesy said had never happened.

Thus I lived with two elderly people who tried to pick logos off my T-shirts, thinking the Polo players were tangles of thread.

I grew sensitive to remarks about a grown man living with his parents, like the character, Robert, on the television show *Everybody Loves Raymond*. I stuck to a routine, going to Starkey Park to practice martial arts in the morning, teaching college in the evening, entering a golf scramble on Saturday mornings and getting a hero's welcome when I returned home with a wad of cash. I cooked Nathan's hotdogs for Stephen and Barbara every Saturday at five o'clock, wondering what other people were doing, wondering if I could survive without a social life.

At times I felt ineffective in coping, but my mission became clearer one day when I read my horoscope in the newspaper: "Your task is to lovingly protect." I took comfort in this even though the infinitive had been split. I couldn't change the way things were headed, but I could offer support and from time to time provide an element of security. I thought, you can forget about being the same person as you were coming into this. You won't be.

One evening after dark I joined my parents in the living room. Stephen sat in his recliner, its broken springs ready to lacerate anyone who reached under it. Wearing a bathrobe, Barbara stood at the kitchen counter, sorting and arranging pills. I sat on the sofa and saw Barbara standing in the half-light by the counter.

She suddenly turned to face us.

"I'm dizzy," she said.

She grabbed her groin area and reached out with one hand to hold the counter. She stepped forward unsteadily, sank into her recliner, and put her head back.

"Are you alright, Mom?" I said.

My mother's eyes closed. The muscles in her face and neck began to clench and contort. I knelt in front of her and touched her hands. They were wet and cold. She was gripping the arms of her recliner with all her might. Sweat coated her face. The muscles in her jaw and cheek rippled and pulled her face out of shape.

"Can you hear me, Mom?" I said.

She didn't say anything.

I remembered Barbara describing Stephen's face as "slumping" when he had suffered a stroke in a theatre in Aruba. I knew without a doubt that Barbara was having a stroke.

Stephen said from his chair, "That wasn't good."

"No," I said, "I think Mom is having a stroke. Shouldn't we call an ambulance?"

Stephen stood up. He came halfway across the living room.

"Mom," he said. "Mom, do you want to go to the hospital? Or do you want to go to your room?"

"My room," she said, barely conscious.

We supported her between us, leading her to the bed. We laid her down with her head supported by pillows. I shoved her body and legs toward the center of the bed and pulled the covers over her. Her face was pale. Large droplets of sweat pocked her forehead.

I wanted to feel her temperature and to wipe away the sweat, so I reached my hand out.

"Don't wake her up!" Dad said.

The moment I touched her, she awakened and looked around. I noticed color coming back into her face.

"Bring me some saltine crackers and some ginger ale," she said, as if nothing unusual was going on.

I went to the kitchen and got the crackers and the drink and brought them to her. She began to eat the crackers and to sip the ginger ale.

A couple days later Barbara was out front pruning dead leaves in her flower garden. I told her what had happened the other night. I explained that I thought she had suffered a stroke and that Dad and I had put her to bed and had not sent her to the hospital. I wanted to know what she thought about it—if what we did had been the right thing to do.

"Maybe I did have a stroke," Barbara said. "I guess I could have gone to the hospital. But you never know when it might just be your time."

I had lived with my parents over a year when I began to hear my name, "Chris!", spoken in the middle of the night in an urgent voice that woke me up. The voice was compelling, as if someone were standing outside the open door of my bedroom, yet I wasn't sure whose voice it was, if it were my mother's or my father's voice or another voice made up of both of them.

I bolted awake and sat up in bed, amazed. I leaned forward with the sheet over my legs and listened in the darkness of the house.

WEDDING RINGS

The summer kept producing days of glorious heat and teeming plant growth. The previous March I had cut my parents' allamanda vine down to a stump. By June it had made a complete comeback putting forth yellow trumpets and again needing to be pruned and shaped.

On Wednesdays I grilled ham steaks covered with barbeque sauce the way Barbara told me to: on low heat, keeping the meat soft so Stephen could chew it. Barbara made potato salad and set out plates of olives, cheese, tomato, carrots and celery. She cut the ham on Stephen's plate into bite-sized pieces before sitting down at the table.

I tried to keep the conversation upbeat, to make no mention of Parkinson's, glaucoma, melanoma or hypertension. I told them that the allamanda native to Florida was a vine like ours, while the allamanda bushes that you saw were imported from Brazil.

"When you cut the allamanda vine, a milky fluid comes out that's toxic to humans," I told them, forking a piece of ham. "You have to wear gloves to work on it."

My father replied, "He's not an arborist, even if he does play one on television."

Barbara was sleepy and forgetful. Twice she lost track of her wedding rings, and I was commissioned to find them: once I found them floating in her bed covers, and the other time I found them under the bed, the two rings taped together.

Stephen had bought Barbara a new wedding band after she slammed her finger on a sliding glass door. Her finger had swollen, and she had to have her old ring cut off. The new ring was a simple gold band like the original wedding ring, and she wore it taped with white adhesive tape to a diamond ring that had belonged to her mother, Rena Moore.

On Sundays they ate fast food, with Barbara making a run in the car to Arby's for roast beef sandwiches and to McDonald's for french fries and the strawberry milk shakes that Stephen wanted. She made her fast food run after the end of the Buccaneers football game.

I went with her. The first time we went to Arby's, Barbara placed her order through the intercom, then pulled up to the window and paid for the food. As soon as she received her change, she told me, "Well, there's nothing more for me to do here," and put the car in gear and drove off.

This happened several times. I tried to write it off to nervousness. I began making the fast food runs by myself. Traffic was busy.

The sun-suffused days slowly faded into quiet autumn. I came and went from the golf course to school and home again as my mother and father drifted unconscious in their recliners. Barbara slept for hours during the day, and Stephen had to bark at her from his recliner to wake her up.

I taught classes on the third floor of a new classroom building at PHCC. Before class I climbed the outside stairwell to the third story and gazed out across the green textured carpet of treetops, the oaks and pine, looking for oncoming clouds, enjoying the drama of faraway bolts of lightning, judging exactly where Stephen and Barbara's subdivision lay hidden, thinking it was beyond my comprehension that my mother and my father were out there, only a mile away, sitting in their living room, Dad giving the channel selector a workout, their TV blaring, with Mom solving word puzzles or dozing in her chair.

At Sam's Club, Barbara pushed a huge blue plastic shopping cart through the aisles. In an abundance of caution, she yielded the right-of-way to any and every shopper in her path. She waited for people to pass who were not even coming near us. After we loaded cases of lemon-flavored green tea and laundry soap into the blue basket, the cart was too heavy for Barbara to start it in motion.

In the world of Sam's Club, in the vast parking lot and the wide store aisles, Barbara now occupied the lowest rung of the ladder. She was the feeblest person, the least aggressive and least assertive person in Sam's Club. On a given day, that distinction has to belong to someone, and the time had come for that distinction to belong to my mother.

I wanted to go with her, but if I wasn't at home, Barbara drove herself. The holidays were approaching, and she purchased a carton of Beck's beer for me but left it in a shopping cart in the parking lot.

I overheard Barbara making a telephone call to Sam's Club, asking if anyone had "turned in a box of beer." No one had.

Barbara bought a ring as a Christmas present for Andrea. Before she giftwrapped the ring, she tried it on and showed it to Stephen. She pulled her taped-together wedding rings off her finger. She did this standing in front of Stephen as he sat in his recliner, and she placed her rings on the glass top of a sturdy rattan coffee table from the Philippines.

She couldn't remember whether she had dropped the rings, put them in her pocket or set them down somewhere, but she couldn't find them. She asked me to look for them, and I scoured the area but came up empty.

My mother was a brave woman. When she had first told me about her outbreak of melanoma, I remember her saying, "I'm not afraid."

I drove them to Publix supermarket—with Stephen coming along, I supposed, to offer moral support. Barbara was quiet and concerned but uncomplaining. I remember looking at Barbara's face, sensing her preoccupation, and thinking, *This is an eighty-one year old woman who is saddened and hurt because she has lost her wedding rings, her most treasured possessions.*

The three of us knew, as a family, that there wasn't going to be any light-heartedness, any levity, while those rings were missing.

Barbara didn't say much about it. She took care of her husband and went about her business, but she was still yearning for the rings. Two days later, mid-morning, I saw Barbara stoop over in her straight-legged fashion and lift the skirt of fabric attached to the couch and take a look under it. I knew immediately that we could trust an old lady's intuition. She had stopped to look there because that was in fact where she had lost her rings.

I got down on the floor and searched, my face an inch from the carpet.

Sure enough, the cream-colored leg of the heavy rattan table had carved deeply into the rug and an object had fitted itself into the crevasse, slipping almost entirely out of sight. I pulled it out: a thin gold ring fastened with smudged adhesive tape to a tiny band of diamonds.

"Look," I said to Mom.

She was seated in her recliner. She saw what was resting in my palm, and she reached for it, her fingers digging with strength into the hollow of my palm as she took the rings.

"Daddy! Chrissy found my rings!" she said.

"Good, by golly!" Stephen said, relieved, from the other room.

That evening, as I headed out the door to go to PHCC, Barbara came up to me.

"Here, this is for what you did," she said.

Into my hand she tucked a folded twenty-dollar bill.

After a trip to Sam's Club, we packed cases of drinks and bulky items like watermelon and cantaloupe into the refrigerator in the garage and carried the rest of the loot into the house.

My mother and I sat down in the living room. Then my father came in from the garage and stood next to the table in the dining area, not far from the sets of blinds that he opened every morning.

My mother, surprised at something, pointed past me into the space between my father and the master bedroom.

"There. I saw her walk past," she said.

"Who?" I asked.

"One of Daddy's great-aunts. She came right out of his body and kept going and went into the bedroom wearing a coat and a hat."

I recalled the pictures of the great-aunts at Seymour Lake. Bean, Barry,

Drew, if those were their family names, ladies of a bygone age, a bygone era, somehow making their presence known.

"Which one was it?" I said.

Barbara said, "I don't know. I didn't know her well, only when Daddy was a little boy."

Barbara had seen ladies standing in our yard and within the house near the front door. She had seen her mother, Rena Moore, in the same fashion, always attired in coat and hat.

Several times Barbara had seen our neighbor, Joann Chassey, out on the sidewalk, looking at our house, bending at the waist with her finger pressed to her lips saying, "Shhh."

DIGNITY NETWORK

———— ··◈·· ————

Two men from North Meadowlawn Funeral Home came over, invited by Barbara and Stephen after the men had given a lunch presentation at the Veterans Administration. I was fortunate enough to be home to see these men in action. The men were slick, Southern, friendly. They both wore white shirts with neckties, pants with suspenders, and neither of them wore a jacket. Stephen showed them the pictures of the USS *Ray* on display in the bedroom. They greatly admired the sub and praised Stephen's service to our nation.

The sales pitch was supposed to climax with Barbara and Stephen purchasing a prearranged funeral—the urns, the flowers, the rest of the decor, the pastor, the speech, all sorted out ahead of time. This arrangement would eliminate the need for members of the family, like me, they pointed out, nodding in my direction, to make difficult decisions while in a saddened, emotional state.

Barb and Steve didn't want to buy a prearranged funeral. They said they hardly knew anyone in Florida. After they died, their family would most likely hold a service in Vermont. All they wanted to purchase now was their cremation.

The men were berserk, frustrated. They'd just come from another old couple's house nearby where the old folks had said the exact same thing: no $10,000 funeral, thank you, just the cremation.

They managed to sell Barbara and Stephen an "away from home" coverage option: If you died while away on a trip, they took your body to the nearest Dignity Network provider to be cremated. Then they shipped the cremains wherever you wanted.

This option proved to be a bone of contention because Barbara and Stephen decided to cancel "away from home" coverage after a few payments, precipitating many dunning calls to the house from the Dignity Network.

I offered to get on the phone with the Dignity Network rep and tell her we weren't paying, but Stephen told me to stay out of it.

A GOOD NAIL

꧁ ꧂

Barbara now had trouble following a recipe, a disconcerting development for someone who had for sixty-two years made succulent meat loaves and French onion soup, proudly setting these foods before her husband at the dinner table. Her pies, cakes, and cookies, of which I was a major consumer, were her trademarks. At one point, when she talked with me about her memory loss, I had joked, saying, "Just don't forget how to bake a cake."

News came of the decline of Barbara's friend, Edna Williams. Her husband, Billy, called the house to tell her and Stephen about it. Billy was the submarine vet who had served with Stephen aboard the *Ray*.

Edna William's dementia had developed with inexorable quickness. At first she had become jealous and irrational, prone to outbursts of all varieties. At a family gathering in Indiana, she had become indignant and uncooperative, imagining people were insulting her, and she drove herself back to Jacksonville, Florida, before the rest of the family knew she was missing.

Billy told Barbara that Edna had been institutionalized. Billy still visited her, but she no longer recognized him.

This was terrible news for Barbara. In Edna's story, I'm sure my mother heard the echo of her own loss of certainty and sanity.

Although she was greatly saddened by Edna Williams' breakdown, what was to follow—the loss of Aunt Tally and Uncle Bud Nealy— pushed my mother over the edge. Aunt Tally and my Aunt Jeanne were sisters from the Lewis family. Bud and Tally were looked after by Jeanne's daughter, Pamela, and Pamela's husband, John Lestage. Pam and John lived in South Carolina but came to Florida every winter.

Pam said that to talk to Bud and Tally on the phone, you would think they weren't experiencing any problem at all. When Pamela and John visited in 2007, they found Bud and Tally in poor health. They were in a state of mental denial, subsisting on a diet of ice cream bars. Pam and John found Tally drinking Bloody Marys in her living room chair while Bud sat across the room in his recliner, incontinent.

First, Uncle Bud passed away. Then Tally.

After Tally passed away, my mother was in shock. She went about the house in a trance, not saying a word about Bud and Tally.

One night we were preparing a dinner of leftovers, and Barbara got mixed up with too many things on the stove. I told her to relax and have a drink while I finished cooking. That meant monitoring the chicken and pot roast leftovers and putting a tray of frozen French fries into the oven.

Mom sat in her recliner drinking for a minute. Then she came back into the kitchen and asked to sample the French fries. I told her the French fries had only been in the oven for two minutes, so they were still frozen.

She insisted on trying them. She had a faraway look in her eyes. She lifted several cold French fries to her mouth and chewed them, telling me how scrumptious they were.

After washing the dishes, I opened a drawer in the kitchen and found a package of romaine hearts neatly rubber-banded and tucked next to the telephone book.

I picked up the romaine hearts and showed them to Stephen.

"Throw them away," he said.

In the days to follow, I tailed Mom around the house—when I was there—shutting off water faucets that she left running in the kitchen while she went to the garage and foraged in the refrigerator.

Barbara had forgotten how to preheat the oven. She asked me before each meal how I thought we should prepare the food. I was the go-to guy for advice now. She used to do that kind of thing—openly ask me for advice—outside the presence of my father, but no longer.

We moved the furniture to have the carpets cleaned. Chairs perched on the beds, and the recliners sat out in the tiled Florida room. We walked through the house in plastic slippers for a day until the carpet dried. According to me and my father, Barbara wasn't supposed to move anything by herself. She tried to lift a ladder back chair off her bed, though, and a chair rung struck her shin. From this bump grew a large, purple bruise.

As she sat in her recliner applying ice to her shin, we watched blood fill the bruise forming a hematoma the size of an Idaho potato, if the potato were sliced in half and mounted on her leg.

We took her to the ER at Community Hospital, where it was determined that she should have the hematoma treated by her regular doctor.

Barbara's physician, Dr. Ehab Michael, was out of the office on a two-month visit to Israel, so we went to see Dr. Aziz Al'KaFaji, who covered for Dr. Michael and whose office was next door to Dr. Michael's in the medical suite.

Dr. Al'KaFaji was not equipped to remove a hematoma of this size, so we went back to Community Hospital where Barbara was admitted and had the procedure done.

The nursing staff had never seen a hematoma as huge as this one, and they called other nurses and physicians into Barbara's room to see it.

Stephen wanted to wait there while they removed the hematoma. We sat for seven hours in back-breaking chairs in the lobby of the hospital without knowing there was a comfortable lounge upstairs with free coffee and snacks for the families of patients.

I was humiliated.

"I wish I'd known how long this was going to take," I said, "so I could make plans."

"What plans?" Stephen said.

"To read some student papers," I said, "or go home and eat lunch."

The upshot was that home health nurses began arriving at the house with a bewildering lack of regularity.

During the initial assessment conducted at our breakfast table, the nurse asked Barbara if there were any stressful elements in her life.

She whispered, "My son," pointing over her shoulder, her thumb jabbing in the direction of my bedroom. I was standing directly behind her.

This was the day after the potato-sized hematoma was removed. She had left her dentures at the hospital, so I drove back to retrieve them, taking Dad with me.

"We'll be gone for a while, Mom, so you can talk to the nurses about anything you want to," I said.

Dad and I went back to Community Hospital and hung out drinking coffee in the cafeteria.

The home health nurse took over the glass-topped table, spread out her papers and organized the rest of her day while taking calls on her cell phone. She entered notes into a red folder, describing Barbara as mentally disorganized and unable to follow a train of thought.

A sponge was tightly bandaged on the site of her hematoma. The sponge was attached by a tube to a device that sucked moisture out of the sponge. The device was the size of an early model cell phone or a reel-to-reel tape recorder and was just as heavy and came with a sling for carrying.

Over the following weeks, several nurses took turns changing the bandage on Mom's leg. Their performances varied considerably: some taped the bandage too tightly; others didn't dare remove the old bandage and left without doing anything.

A male nurse took me aside wanting me to know that my mother and father were not safe in the house by themselves.

"What does he do?" he asked, nodding in the direction of my father, who had walked past us to to empty a glass of ice cubes into the kitchen sink.

I thought the male nurse had noticed Stephen's eye, opaque with silvery glaucoma.

"He doesn't see well," I said.

The nurse was in disbelief when I told him that my mother still drove the car, telling me that the notes in the red folder included an indication of psychosis.

Although Barbara had the leg injury and the heavy device to carry, it was Stephen who was acting morose. He sat at the breakfast table with a drawn expression as Barbara read the headlines in the newspaper, her bandaged leg attached to a ball and chain.

I got ready to drive Barbara to a doctor's appointment. She came out to the garage carrying the heavy device. The mood was quarrelsome. Stephen stood in the garage wearing his bathrobe, waiting for us to leave.

Barbara opened the passenger side door. She looked back at Stephen.

"You're so mean to me," she sobbed.

As Barbara climbed into the front seat, the car door sprang back a few inches and struck her in the forehead.

"You klutz!" Stephen said, watching us from the embrasure of the door to the laundry room.

Those were his words of encouragement to his wife.

Fierce rainstorms barrel through Florida during the summer, drenching the lawns, coating patio furniture with a film of dirt, filling the retention ponds, washing away chunks of the asphalt roads.

I cleaned dirt and mildew off a set of white vinyl chairs on the front porch. Seeking approval, I brought this chore to Barbara's attention. She lowered the magazine she was reading.

"Well, I'm glad you're doing something to make up for all the hot water you've been using," she said. "Our water bill was over $60 last month."

"I take quick showers," I said. "I'm not the one who walks off leaving the water running."

I washed the vinyl ceiling of the Florida room. The job took two rainy mornings, working on a stepladder, pressing rags into the corrugated vinyl. As I worked, Barbara read to Stephen at the breakfast table, her hematoma slowly healing, the two of them visible to me through the sliding glass doors.

There was a songbird calendar that hung in the garage with dates circled indicating all the "blue bag" days when a truck came to pick up bottles and cans to be recycled. Dates were circled every other week on the entire calendar, but the dates circled were not the correct ones: in fact, the recycling truck came on the Tuesdays that were not circled.

It didn't matter.

The problem with the songbird calendar, the "blue bag" calendar, was that it hung on a white brad that sometimes slipped into the wallboard so it appeared to be lost. When this happened, I dug the brad out of the wall with my fingernails and hung the calendar, changing the page to the next songbird.

Once Barbara's leg had healed, she was in motion again.

As I washed some pots and pans one evening, Barbara came in from the garage where she and Stephen were working. She carried a hammer. She opened the drawer where I had found the romaine hearts and started fishing around in the drawer.

"Where can I find a good nail?" she asked.

"What do you need it for?" I said.

"That bird calendar keeps coming down, and I'm going to fix it."

"I can get that nail out," I said. "It slips into the wall."

"I just need to get my hands on a good nail."

"There's a box of nails on the shelf above your golf clubs," I said.

Barbara went back to the garage. I dried another dish and followed her. As I opened the door to the garage, I heard a thump as she drove the nail through the body of the Eastern bluebird.

She went back into the house. My father and I stood in the garage, looking at the calendar nailed through to the wall.

"Can we book her a room in the nuthouse?" I said.

"She's not going anywhere," he told me. "She's here to stay, come hell or high water. I don't know what your plans are, but she's here to stay, by George."

"Well, I'm not staying," I said. "I'm leaving."

Dad looked at me. He didn't say anything. I didn't know what he could see through his reverse tunnel vision and a cornea that looked like dead keratin. A diseased, eighty-two year old man was standing in the garage of a house that had been a blessing for sixteen years but was now an enigma, and I had tried to hurt him. I gave it my best parting shot. I pulled out all the stops on my need for payback for years of perceived belittlement, lack of recognition, and mistrust.

Before he started serving as a U.S. Customs Officer, my father had worked as a State Trooper in Vermont for twenty years. One snowy night in Newport, I came back to our family's house on Eastern Avenue and stomped my boots and brushed heavy flakes of snow off my jacket. My mother greeted me in the kitchen.

She said, "Daddy says a group of boys threw snowballs at the cruiser, and he thinks you were one of them. Were you?"

"No," I said. "I'm not that stupid."

A small town in Vermont had only one State Trooper, one cruiser, in town, if that. Did my father think I was so numb that I would bomb his cruiser with ice balls?

My worst memory, though, involved the Newport Country Club where my father was a member. One summer day, my cousin Kit, David's brother, was visiting from East Islip, Long Island. We played twenty-seven holes of golf that day, finishing after all the other golfers had left.

We had gotten into trouble with the president of the golf club, who was playing in a foursome behind us. The club president struck an errant shot that almost hit me, and I swore at him.

After we finished our front nine, the greens keeper told us to leave the premises. Kit led me into the grill at the clubhouse where the club president was having lunch, and he begged the club president's pardon for our behavior. In a weak moment, the club president told us to go ahead and finish our back nine. So we did.

When we were finished playing the twenty-seven holes, Kit and I walked back down Pine Hill toward town, the hillside bathed with sunshine, the City of Newport lying quaint below us, the sheen of Lake Memphremagog stretching toward Canada. It was so quiet you felt you could lean forward and cup your ear to hear ninth-inning cheers all the way from Fenway Park or feel shock waves from the five o'clock thunder in Yankee Stadium. But Kit and I became part of the lore of that summer in a way that we didn't anticipate or welcome.

Coming up the hill was George Shover, a wiry guy with greasy black hair combed into a DA, a reputed troublemaker and an outsider at my high school.

We didn't know for a fact what George did that evening, but that night someone flooded and gouged several greens on the golf course. They had opened some spigots and flooded the greens and then had taken a rake from a sand trap and had gouged the greens and ruined them.

Kit and I were the last people to be seen at the course that night, and since we had already gotten into trouble, we were accused of destroying those golf greens.

This was brought up to my father's mortification at a membership meeting at the country club.

Although I denied doing it, my father bought into the accusations. After that, I stopped playing golf altogether. I attended the University of Vermont and began writing poetry and fiction. I didn't pick up a golf club again for fifteen years until I was married to a woman whose parents were avid golfers.

Somehow this thread of past crimes, this trail of crumbs, was reconstituted as I talked to Barbara in the kitchen, when Stephen abruptly cut the sound on the TV set to see if we were talking about him. I had told her that Kit and I had never done it, had never destroyed those golf greens.

"Daddy, did you hear what Chris said?" she called out. "He said they didn't do it!"

There was joy in her voice as she called to my father, as if this decades-old sin had been freshly weighing on their minds. I looked with curiosity at my father as he absorbed what my mother was saying. He wore his usual stony expression but seemed to understand what she meant.

It was too late for a scene of reconciliation. My father had lived half a lifetime with this alleged tarnish upon our reputations. A father bore the burden of the flaws and errors of his children, if he had knowledge of them, and carried the knowledge to his deathbed.

Despite our past misunderstandings, I felt that I had to help my parents cope with the challenges of their last years. Not doing so would have been a terrible lost opportunity. Already divorced, something of a loner, looking into the future, I didn't want to have to second guess any decision regarding my family. I did not want the burden of having avoided them when they needed help, for instance. I wanted to know what was happening to them, and it was in my best interest to see things first hand.

WAR MEDALS

"We never should have moved down here in the first place," Stephen was saying from his recliner. "We never should have come to Florida."

The framed pastel portraits of his three daughters animated the wall of the living room, their high school-aged faces looking healthy and vital.

Our plans to move Stephen and Barbara to a cottage in an assisted living complex in Connecticut were slow in materializing.

"We should have put this house on the market when we had the chance," Barbara said. "The agent said she could sell our house for $215,000."

That offer was made four years ago when the housing market was booming.

"I'm going out," I said. "I'm meeting a friend of mine, Lena, over at Books-A-Million."

I made sure to use Lena's name to suggest her gender. I wanted to eradicate any resemblance to Ray Romano's fictional brother, Robert, a character on *Everybody Loves Raymond*. I needed to prove that I didn't share Robert's dilemmas and frustrations.

"I'll be back in a few hours," I said on my way out the door.

"Well, have fun," Barbara said.

I drove along Embassy Boulevard toward the disc of sun dropping in a nectarine haze over the Gulf, wondering how this date would turn out.

Lena was named after Lena Horne. Lena said we had a lot in common; we both loved jazz and literature. She was a Native American with a friendly personality and long dark hair and caramel-colored skin. Frankly, I was looking forward to getting my hands on her. One rainy night, she gave me a ride in her car just to the other side of campus, and before I got out of the car, I managed to brush against her soft and creamy bare shoulder.

I waited on the sidewalk outside Books-A-Million until I was sweaty and it was obvious Lena was going to be really late or wasn't coming. I called her. She explained that her girlfriend had a flat tire and that she had to go pick her up. I didn't ask Lena why she had not called earlier to tell me, and I didn't ask the other questions that swirled in my mind. We rescheduled, and I drove home.

I parked the Nissan under the rustling Queen palms at the Keiths' house.

As I opened the door to the living room, Barbara looked up from her book of word puzzles. Stephen turned down the volume of the TV.

"What happened?" Barbara asked.

"Lena's girlfriend had a flat tire," I said. "She had to go help her."

Stephen and Barbara looked at each other.

"Well, I'm sorry that didn't work out for you," Barbara said.

"I'm meeting her over there next week," I said, clawing for a shred of self-esteem, suddenly feeling awkward in my clean, casual dating clothes.

I went into my room and changed into beaten-up khaki shorts and a Polo T-shirt. I surfed the internet for a couple of hours then went to sleep.

John and Reni Chamberlain flew in from California in June of 2008. John Chamberlain needed to have a medical procedure performed on his throat, and he came to Tampa because the best throat surgeon in the nation was here.

John Chamberlain was a legend to me, although I had never met the man. All the stories I'd heard about him came from the remote past. In fact, I'd never envisioned him as anything but a young boy.

Chamberlain's mother was my grandmother's sister. When he was a child, Chamberlain had lived with my father for several years. Chamberlain and his mother were taken into my grandmother's house after Chamberlain's father had abandoned them.

So they lived together as boys, and I speculated that some jealousy on my father's part had developed. My father was several years older than Chamberlain and had gone into the Navy first, joined the War in the Pacific, and become a Torpedoman's Mate Second Class. Chamberlain, who enlisted in the Navy years later, advanced to the rank of Commander of a nuclear submarine. I don't know whether or not this was the source of my father's jealousy, or whether something else happened to cause friction, and in fact I truly don't know that any jealousy ever existed.

We waited for the Chamberlains to arrive. When Reni Chamberlain came out of the sunlight into the shade of the garage and saw me, she stopped in her tracks. She told me that I looked exactly like her son, Christopher. Both her sons had been successful Navy pilots. Christopher would have been my age if he had lived—had he not killed himself.

The coincidence was that Reni and Barbara each had sons named Stephen and Christopher, and each had a son who took his life: Barbara's son, Stephen, and Reni's son, Christopher.

We stood in the master bedroom below the pictures of USS *Ray* breaching the surface of a surly, sepia ocean. We were looking at a display of military medals earned long ago by my Grandfather Keith, and by my uncles and my father. Among the old medals was a beautiful new addition: the Philippine Republic Presidential Unit Citation dating back to 13 May 1948, given in recognition of the *Ray's* effort in supplying the resistance movement and in transporting intellectuals and escaped prisoners of war from the Philippines while the country was under Japanese occupation.

Stephen had recently received the ribbon and letter of commendation. He couldn't have been more proud. It was a great moment of recognition for Stephen in a life subdued by muscular stiffness, bodily pain, blindness, hallucination and depression.

We stood looking at the foreign citation ribbon, a rarity among American servicemen. I had been shown the medals in this frame when I was child. They were kept upstairs in my grandparents' house in a room which served a dual purpose as my grandmother's knitting room and as a place for gun racks packed with my grandfather's muskets and shotguns.

When I first saw the display of medals, it had included a silver icon of a nuclear submarine pinned over on the right side. That silver icon belonged to John Chamberlain. The icon of the nuclear sub hadn't been in the display for decades. I don't know when it was removed, the circumstances of that removal, whether it had been returned to John Chamberlain, or any other details.

The Chamberlains and the Keiths drank and reminisced. Chamberlain was a successful man, the President of the golf club on the naval base in California where he had been based. By late afternoon, though, he felt worn out from the surgery on his throat and needed to drive Reni back to their motel.

I took their snapshot in the Florida room by the orchids, not knowing it would be the penultimate picture to be taken of my father. In the picture, Dad wears a frozen, unhappy expression, one hand in his shorts pocket, the tattoo of a three-masted schooner visible on his forearm. Barbara holds Stephen's other hand, her bruised hand and bandaged arm emerging from an attractive, patterned sleeve. John Chamberlain has removed his neck brace for purposes of the group photo. Reni looks up at Chamberlain rather than at the camera.

That was the day before Dad went to the hospital, never to return to his home on Pineneedles Drive.

DAD

I left the bedroom door open while I slept so the ceiling fans could do their work and circulate air through my end of the house.

At four o'clock I opened my eyes and saw my mother standing by my door in the semi-dark, saying, "Chris, Daddy's throwing up blood and it's coming out his pooper. We have to take him to the hospital."

I got up and pulled on a pair of shorts. I knew the moment had come that fulfilled the purpose of my coming to Florida and justified my moving in with them—the moment that I wanted neither my mother nor my father to face by themselves.

I went into the master bedroom and found Dad lying half on and half off the bed, bare chested, with an unbuttoned pair of blue plaid shorts around his hips.

"Oh, boy," he said when he saw me. "Jesus."

I got a towel and held it to his mouth as he threw up more blood. The blood was black and thick with mucus.

Mom showed her grace under pressure by calling an ambulance, speaking into the phone with total lucidity, reading the 10435 Pineneedles Drive address from a slip of note paper she had written out.

When I first saw how much blood Dad had lost into the toilet and sink, I thought he was going to die. Then I realized that if the aneurysm in his chest had burst, he would not be conscious, and my fears subsided.

EMTs arrived at the front door. They pushed a gurney into the bedroom leaving black wheel tracks on the off-white carpet. The EMTs were down-to-earth and professional as they took care of Dad. Off he went into the night. A few minutes later Mom and I followed in Dad's Mercury Sable.

Mom gave me Dad's billfold to hold onto. We got to the ER at Community Hospital, showed Dad's insurance cards, and got him admitted.

He was lying on a bed in a large bay partitioned into little rooms by anemic blue curtains pulled back and forth as more people were brought in. Mom and I sat beside Dad's bed on metal folding chairs on a concrete floor.

Dad was conscious and stable.

"I thought I had come to the end of the world," he said.

Someone placed a can of soda next to Dad's bed; otherwise, no one looked at him or checked his condition. It seemed to me that hours were passing, so I spoke to the doctor on duty. He took notes on a computer as I told him that Dad had a history of bleeding ulcers, and I suggested that that might be the problem.

Mom and I sat with Dad until six o'clock when Dad told us to go home.

I cleaned the toilet bowl full of blood in the master bathroom while Mom scrubbed the carpet next to the bed.

We went back to Community Hospital a few hours later. Dad had been placed in a room on the first floor. Still no doctors had attended to him. No procedure had been scheduled. Not realizing that Dad had lost three units of blood, I called my sister, Joanna, and told her that Dad's condition was not life-threatening.

After supper, Mom and I made our third visit of the day to Community Hospital. We went to the room on the first floor, but Dad wasn't there. Dr. Patel, a gastroenterologist, was standing in the hallway talking with Dr. Shielah Drevon, Dad's regular physician.

When Dr. Patel saw Mom, he stopped her and told her that Dad had lost more blood and had almost died. He was now upstairs in intensive care.

Dr. Patel was finally ready to perform a procedure on Dad. He was going to staple closed a gaping ulcer in Dad's stomach, probably the result of Dad's daily ingestion of low dose Bayer aspirin. It was seven in the evening, and I had told the doctor in the ER about Dad's history of ulcers at four-thirty that morning.

I realized that I had left my cell phone at home, but I wanted it now in case something happened to Dad during this procedure and I had to call my sisters. I asked Mom to stay in the living room-like lounge for families of people in the IC while I drove home and got my cell phone. It was only a ten minute drive each way.

When I got to the car I noticed a smear of yellow paint on the driver's side door where someone had had struck our car while pulling out of their parking space. I drove home and retrieved the cell phone but felt that I was away from Mom for too long.

I parked the car again and got out. I found Mom wandering under the portico in front of the hospital. When she saw me, she was upset, saying she never wanted me to help her again.

I tried to get Mom to come into the hospital with me while I got a briefing from Dr. Patel. She told me Patel had already talked to her about it, and she refused to go back in.

I went back to the IC by myself. Dr. Patel updated me on the procedure and gave me a color print of the ulcer in Dad's stomach.

I shouldn't have left Mom by herself. I had expected the stapling of the stomach ulcer to take longer, and this erroneous expectation had led to my blunder.

The following morning we had to pick up Mom's vacuum cleaner from Hudson Vacuum before we drove to the hospital. Mom tried to give me directions, but I didn't understand them. I asked her again where we were supposed to turn off Little Road. We were standing in the kitchen at the counter.

"I don't know how you could do such a hateful thing," she said, "as to try to confuse me."

"I'm not trying to confuse you," I said. "It's twenty miles round trip. I just want to know where I'm going."

In hindsight, I should have searched for Hudson Vacuum online. I remembered the place once we got there. It was tucked into a cyclone-fenced lot near the Gulf, not far from where Mom and Dad lived when they first moved to Florida, in the bad little town of Hudson.

After we picked up the vacuum cleaner, we drove ten miles down

U.S. 19 to Community Hospital. In the IC unit Dad was sitting up in bed, a nurse feeding him tempting spoonfuls of apple sauce and sips of chocolate milk. He told me to find him an attorney. There was going to be an arraignment tomorrow, and he needed a lawyer to represent him. Almost laughing, I asked what the arraignment was for. Prior to his career as a Customs Officer, Dad had served in the Vermont State Police for twenty years, so he knew what an arraignment was all about.

I wanted to figure out if there was something out of Dad's past that might be bothering him. I wondered if the trauma from his loss of blood had unearthed concerns of his that had long been buried. I asked Dad more about it, but my probing led nowhere.

Joanna caught a flight from Massachusetts and joined us. After a few days, Dad was feeding himself pudding and was able to leave the IC unit and return to a room on the first floor of the hospital. There, Dr. Patel told Dad that he needed to battle to stay alive. He had to try to exercise by rising out of bed and getting into a chair, then getting back in bed, and doing it again as many times as he could. Mom exhorted Dad to make this effort.

It seemed unfair to let three units of blood out of someone then tell them they were in a war zone, but that's what happened.

Again, Dad urged me to find an attorney so he could be ready for the arraignment.

"You take care of your mother," he told me as we were leaving.

At home, Mom confided to Joanna and me that on occasion she had seen Dad give up trying. I didn't know exactly what she referred to by give up. It was something out of their shared history, and I never found out what she meant.

I heard Mom tell Joanna, "Christopher is trying to take over the house."

I don't know when she first formulated that thought. Dad had only been gone for a couple of days. I had always shown deference to them, never making unilateral decisions. I would even let them know when I was about to put in new log edger around the flower beds or when I was going to trim the bird-of-paradise.

At the hospital, not knowing what else I could do, I applied Reiki healing over Dad as he lay sleeping. When he was awake, Joanna swabbed the gummy secretions from Dad's eyes and cleaned out his mouth with a mint-flavored sponge pad on a stick.

Complicating matters was the swallow study Dr. Patel had ordered. Just at the point when Dad was able to feed himself again, Dr. Patel discovered that Dad was aspirating his food, and Patel deemed swallowing to be unsafe. Our family knew about the aspiration. For years Mom had risen from her place at the supper table to pound Dad's back when he began to choke. Every mealtime, Dad's eyes watered and his nose began to run, indications that he was aspirating food. At the table, he dabbed away at his eyes and nose with a handkerchief.

Dr. Patel ordered a G-tube to be inserted into Dad's stomach to prevent the aspiration.

At first, my sister, Andrea, questioned the appropriateness of the G-tube, reminding us that Dad had a living will and was not supposed to be kept alive artificially, but we didn't know if the G-tube contradicted the will and went ahead with it.

Dad needed rehab, PT, skilled nursing care above and beyond what could be provided in his home. At least by us.

We looked at a list of nursing homes, and Joanna picked one that Mary Keith, who worked as a volunteer at Bayonet Point Hospital, had not crossed off the list with an X as being inadequate.

Dad's admittance to Windsor Woods fell on the Fourth of July weekend. Joanna met with the office manager and signed paperwork, coming back to the room to explain the do-not-resuscitate provision, the DNR, to which Dad agreed.

In Dad's room, I moved the bulky visitor's chair from the corner so that Mom could sit close to him. I adjusted the air conditioning unit to its quietest setting and picked up crayon drawings from the dingy linoleum tiles. I glanced at June's activity calendar taped on the wall and sat down on the bed by the door.

Dad needed to urinate, but he couldn't manage the bottle that was left in the bed for him. Joanna and I tried to get Mom to place the bottle into the correct position, but she could not do it in time, saying she didn't know how a man went to the bathroom.

With the bed wet and Dad himself needing changing, we looked for a CNA but couldn't find one. The nurse's station on our wing was vacant. I went past the closed door of the head nurse's office and went around the corner to look into the dining room which was decorated with bunting but unoccupied.

At last a young male CNA came by the room and promised he would return to help Dad clean up.

"Isn't it awful, Chrissy?" Mom said, once we were home.

Joanna had flown home, and my sister Andrea had joined us. We were distraught. Having seen no nurses and no therapists at Windsor Woods, I was furious, not appreciating the impact of the holiday weekend on their work force. The next couple of days were no better, the bottle for urination panning out to be an utter failure.

"You should see where they had me last night," Dad was telling me. "They kept me in a cellar hole underground. It had a window like this one."

He pointed to the wire-reinforced glass of the room's window. I looked out the window at a bird feeder with no seeds in it and a bird-of-paradise without blossoms.

Removed from the familiarity of his home and the company of his trusted consort, Dad was hit with unimaginable worry. He was down in spirit and not interested in learning to use the channel selector for the television. Mom brought the newspaper to read to Dad as they used to do, yet Dad was not in the mood to hear the headlines, the sports, the funny papers, or pages from the book on submarine warfare that Mom had been reading to him in the comfort of their bed at home.

Following Andrea's visit, my sister Alison flew down from Massachusetts to see Dad. She stayed several days, encouraging Dad to work hard on his therapy. After she went back home, it was just my mother and myself.

Windsor Woods was in Hudson, a ten mile drive from our house. Returning from our morning visit, we brought in the mail, ate lunch, then rested for only minutes before Mom began asking me when we were going back to see Dad.

After July 4, the bustle of the CNAs and therapists rekindled. The corridors of Windsor Woods were packed with aged people ambulating with walkers, some of them with blue straps around their waists linking them to the therapists, some of them managing on their own.

This was no time to be bashful. People practiced treading the corridor with their walkers and turning the wheels of their wheelchairs for all they were worth. The doors of all the rooms were kept open, and people lay within the rooms watching television or resting, sometimes glancing at the people who passed by. On a thickly padded stretcher in the hall, a man lay in a state of catatonia, yet he managed to call for help ceaselessly. Most came and went wordlessly, like throngs of displaced humanity in Dante's Divine Comedy.

Dad's CNA was a kind and strong Cape Verde Island woman named Anna who treated Dad with unceasing generosity. Mom and I were getting our breath, healing some frayed nerves following Dad's catastrophe, and we leaned on Anna to help us regain our confidence and gear up for battle.

"You two together could take care of me," Dad said to me and Mom.

I dreaded the obligation of having to help move Dad's rigid, heavy body to the bathroom or to his bed or to his recliner. I was certain that a disk in my back would explode as I tried to steady his weight in the shower or by the night table. And Mom certainly could not up the ante on her level of care. She had put everything she had into the effort of taking care of Dad, with the appointments, the prescriptions, the eye drops, the bills, and meals.

"You can come home when you can walk again," Mom explained.

She bended down close to him, saying, "Show them what a Keith is made of."

Somehow Dad found strength to start his physical therapy. Once or twice a day Dad made his way down the gray tile of the hallway as he gripped a walker, the blue strap around his waist and a therapist behind him. He wore a navy blue pullover shirt and sweat pants that needed laundering. His rubber-soled moccasins slid along the linoleum tiles. He sometimes stepped on his own feet.

An occupational therapy nurse named Marie worked with Dad with great dedication, making sure "Steve," as she called him, had every opportunity to practice for his upcoming swallow studies. The head nurse told Mom, Alison and me that despite therapy, Dad's swallow protection could not be improved. Parkinson's had already taken its toll.

Dad's wit and satirical attitude won him many admirers among the nursing home staff, but he seemed not to want to interact with other patients. His blindness and an inner reluctance that I cannot explain held him back. He did not engage with the other men there who, like himself, felt imprisoned and commanded their exhausted wives to take them home.

WHERE TO LIVE

———◆———

Windsor Woods Nursing Home was an elongated structure with nurses' stations at the end of both wings. The wings branched into ells that sequestered larger bedrooms that people had set up like apartments. The dining area sat in the middle of the structure like the abdomen of a spider.

"Did you know the other end of this building connects right up with Grammy Keith's house?" Dad said, making a sweeping motion with the back of his hand.

The Keith's house was our primordial family setting in Newport, Vermont, where Dad and his brothers had grown up, where John Chamberlain and his mother had been taken in, where old Nora Honsinger—originally a Keith and taken into the house after her husband died—defeated my brother and sisters in dozens of games of Chinese checkers at a card table set up in the front living room. My older brother said he knew that Nora was cheating us in every game.

"It must have been a dream, Dad," I said, "because Grammy Keith's house is up in Vermont, and we're in Hudson, Florida."

I thought of the "tremulous prism" through which Nabokov said he viewed his past in his memoir, *Speak, Memory*, and of Nabokov's descriptions of the houses of his childhood. I thought that even the corridors of Windsor Woods could lure consciousness back to houses where people had lived out their formative years—back to the ancient places where the saga of self and family had taken root.

Although experts were recommending that one agree with everything a person with dementia might say, I usually told Mom and Dad the plain truth and just stuck to the facts, making no effort to upbraid them.

Dad's dreams amazed and alarmed him. His mental world distorted by Parkinson's, his dreams were more vivid and compelling than everyday life. As a former police officer, his visions were of confinement and persecution. The wire in the window glass made him think he was in prison.

He told me one morning that he had woken up in the bed of a pickup truck in Newport, Vermont.

Mom held my hand as we walked across the black sealant of the parking lot at Windsor Woods as she had done crossing the parking lots of Community Hospital, the Gulfview Mall, Publix, Dr. Michael's office, Radiology Associates, St. Luke's Cataract and Laser Institute, and Sam's Club. For a month we visited Dad twice a day. At first, so much walking made Mom's legs stronger. Her energy level was heightened by her anxiety over Dad's health. She no longer snoozed in her chair for hours on end as she had done prior to this crisis—the way people will do during the onset of their dementia. While Dad had never watched much baseball on television except for the World Series, Mom wanted to watch the Tampa Bay Rays baseball games. She stayed up so late that I found myself wishing she would go to bed.

The debate continued as to whether Mom and I could take care of Dad at home. Other people made suggestions. Joann Chassey, the nurse who lived across the street from us, urged me to let Dad live out his last months in the house that he knew and loved.

Now that Dad's morning hours were taken up with his therapy, Mom and I paid him one long visit every afternoon. I let the two of them talk in private in Dad's room while I went down the wing and through some doors to a shady, screened-in porch. I sat listening to the unending slap of the plastic blades of the ceiling fan. The imperfect and noisy blades of the fan were bound to slap on and on forever, as life was supposed to go on whether you liked it or not.

Asking a nurse to unhook Dad's G-tube, I took him for a spin in his wheelchair. He hadn't been out-of-doors in a month. As the front doors parted and the hot August breeze surged through Dad's hair, he let out a whoop. I pushed his chair along the sidewalk in back of the building and then parked him in the shade of the portico so he could jaw with the cigarette smokers who occupied the benches. One of them was a Gulf War veteran on indefinitely long rehabilitation. I was happy to see Dad interacting with people.

Some of our trips to Windsor Woods were followed up with grocery shopping, so the round trip expedition took a few hours. I urged Mom through the aisles of Publix as she gave many many items their due consideration, reading the label of a new soup that had come out, hefting a large wooden spoon and debating whether we needed it, being tempted by any item that bore the "two for the price of one" sticker.

I prepared our dinners, making fresh salads of romaine hearts and tomatoes, on occasion driving to the clubhouse at River Ridge and getting take-out orders of crab cakes, something Dad would not have allowed in the house. We looked for interesting birds at the bird feeder—of course, there weren't many birds around during the heat of the summer—and we watched deer and turkey crossing the crayon green fifth fairway of the golf course, the same hole where years ago I had thought Dad looked like Arnold Palmer.

I played golf Saturday mornings, but if I wasn't back by one o'clock, Mom drove herself to Windsor Woods, wanting badly to see Dad. I tried to convince her to wait for me to get back so I could give her a lift, but she wouldn't.

The phone rang one Friday evening around six-thirty. It was Dad on the line. He had gotten to the nurses' station and convinced them to let him use the phone to call his wife.

He told Mom that he had been transferred to the "big house," which is how he referred to the Atria chalet across the parking lot, the facility for the care of people with larger budgets and greater insurance coverage. He wanted Mom to meet him over there.

I tried to reason with her.

"Dad is mixed up," I said. "I'm certain that he hasn't been transferred. Atria would cost a lot more money, and we would have to agree to it."

"He wants me to meet him over there. I'm going right now," she said.

"We can visit him tomorrow," I said. "He'll be okay."

I was exhausted, and I refused to drive back to Windsor Woods that

Friday evening. While I watched golf on television, Mom got in the car, carefully backed out of the driveway, and drove off to Windsor Woods to meet Dad.

Before Mom could return home, the nurse called me and reported what had happened. In error, Mom thought that Dad had been given an injection, and because of this, she had gone to the nurses' station and threatened to sue the nursing home. The nurse wanted me to know that no injection had been administered. What Dad had been given was a tranquilizer in tablet form to help reduce his anxiety.

Letting Mom drive the car was in defiance of the recommendations of the home health nurses, yet she drove herself to her hair salon and other nearby places. She had been driving in that area for so many years that I thought she must be on automatic pilot. I was trying not to be pushy and authoritative. I thought that any signs of bossiness would alienate my mother.

On the way to Windsor Woods one rainy evening, though, while straining to get a glimpse of an assisted living facility off to the left, she swiped the bushes in the median on Little Road. When she got back that night and told me about the incident, she handed over the keys to the car on her own, never to drive again.

We had a tour of the Sunshine Christian Home on Whippoorwill Drive in Holiday. As advertised, it was an old folks' home on a quiet street bathed in late summer sunshine. Residents were gathered in a front room with large windowpanes looking out onto a wide porch and a shady front yard. We were introduced to the smiling supportive staff and shown the therapy room and the occupants' bedrooms. When Mom saw the homey room with its double bed, bureaus, and television, she sobbed. The atmosphere was of peaceful, perfect, quiet old age, yet Dad couldn't be admitted there because of his feeding tube.

One stifling hot day, Dad's frustration came to a pitch. I had been out on the screened porch at Windsor Woods, sitting on slightly mildewed furniture, listening to the ceiling fan lap its way into infinity. When I got back to room 207, I saw that Dad was ready to say to hell with it all. Mom was on the verge of tears, and Dad was about to "do something," as he put it.

Exactly what he would do was not clear.

As Mom and I left, I looked back into the room to see Dad stand up out of his wheelchair and start pulling at the G-tube attached to his stomach.

In an effort to interrupt him, I said, "Dad, are you doing something?"

He looked at me blankly.

In the car, Mom was sobbing.

"I can't believe I've just left him to do that," she said.

"To do what?" I asked.

"To kill himself," Mom said.

"Shouldn't we tell someone?" I asked her.

"What would you want," she said, "if it were you? Would you want your friend to try to stop you?"

After we got home and Mom was in her chair, I told her that I was going over to the golf course for a little while.

"Is that how you celebrate?" she said.

"I'm not celebrating," I said.

I wanted to get outside. At the same time, I was self-conscious and guilty about leaving Mom to her thoughts.

We did not know what to do. I believed that Dad was too weak to take his life. There didn't seem to be any way that he could do it.

I waited an hour then asked Mom if she would mind if I went over to River Ridge and played nine holes. The day was humid, the golf course devoid of other players. Around seven o'clock, I called Windsor Woods to see if Dad was alright. He had been given a shower and was resting comfortably in bed.

Over a period of weeks, the process of visiting Dad became exhausting, our stores of physical energy depleted. Mom lost strength in her legs, and one evening she could not stand up from her recliner. She tried to rise several times but couldn't do it even with my help, and she had to rest between each attempt. At last, with both of us staggering, we got her into her bedroom.

We were tired. We scaled back our visits. We visited Dad four or five times a week.

VOICES

---·❖·---

The sunshine was both overpowering and reassuring. We came and went from Windsor Woods, the house, the grocery store. We drove to the Deaf and Hard of Hearing Services of Florida and picked up a voice control telephone with oversized buttons for Mom to use. We stopped at the Pasco County Library to renew Mom's card and to pick out some books from the shelf of new acquisitions. Mom enjoyed her books, but the hardbound copies were too heavy for her to hold, so we returned them.

"Can you hear those voices coming out of the television?" Mom asked the home health nurse as she pointed to the Hitchcock cabinet housing the TV set, which happened to be turned off.

The nurse glanced over at me. Nothing anybody said surprised me anymore, and I told the nurse that I once had a friend who could hear radio signals captured by a filling in his tooth.

Mom believed I had a woman in my room at night. Have no doubt about it—she had heard the sound of a woman enjoying a lovemaking session.

As I emerged from my bedroom where I had been sitting for two hours with my knees up correcting student papers, she told me, "You've been having quite a party in there."

Unfortunately, there had been no party, and there was no woman.

At night, Mom was bothered by lights shining into her bedroom window. Perhaps the beams from the headlamps of the cars turning the corner of Baltusrol and Pineneedles, Mom thought there were people on our lawn aiming flashlights at the house.

I did my best to anticipate disapproval, but it didn't always work.

I felt obligated to help manage Mom's prescription regimen. I'd found six vials of nortriptylene in her drawer, and I was worried. When I mentioned it, Mom was offended. She said she had all those pills due to a mix-up at the pharmacy. For all I knew, she may have been entirely correct.

She stood beside me at the kitchen counter. I sorted one day's dosage of pills into a custard cup and explained the new system to Mom. Her face quivered and got red. She leaned her face close to mine, looking me in the eye, and said, "I hate you."

Mom became distant and less trusting. Except for holding hands while crossing the parking lots, we didn't make much physical contact. One day, though, I felt like giving her a hug—we had been through so much together. I gently stroked her shoulder through the black sweater she was wearing, yet she pulled away from me, saying, "You're petting me like I'm some kind of cat."

I used to sit and watch television after Mom had gone to bed, but I would wait for her to emerge as she invariably did. Wearing a pink nightie and a plastic nightcap, she came out to adjust the thermostat, usually to raise the temperature.

Sometimes her bedroom door would open, and she would just stick her head out and say to me, "Tell the others that they can come in and take a shower any time they want."

By "the others," she meant my sisters, the same ladies whose pastel portraits radiated color from the wall above the couch where I was sitting.

In September, Joanna and Andrea visited to take care of some items of business. They canceled a fistful of Mom's credit cards—the one she regretted losing the most was the red Macy's card—and they took possession of several photo albums.

Joanna bought a hearing aid for Mom. Recently, Mom had spent a thousand dollars on a hearing aid which had failed, and Dad wouldn't let Mom buy another one. I wanted to negotiate a refund with the store where she bought the hearing aid, but Dad told me to stay out of it. The store had gone out of business anyway.

Andrea drove Mom to Attorney Bell's office to obtain a power of attorney over Mom and Dad. Andrea did obtain the power of attorney, but Mom was left thinking that Andrea worked at the attorney's office.

Mom confided in me that Andrea had shouted at her in the car. Moreover, the POA cost over two hundred dollars, and Mom wanted her money back.

After paying Dad a visit, we ate lunch at Fatty n Mabel's on the river. We sat on the deck over the brackish water, melting in the heat. I threw fish food into the water while we waited, interminably, for our sandwiches to be ready.

Later I suggested that we take a ride to Starkey Park to look at the oak trees, but Mom refused, saying that somehow Daddy would find out we had done something fun together, which would hurt his feelings.

Mom had trouble with my sisters' names and identities. After she had been talking with Joanna in the screened-in Florida room, she came into the living room and asked me who she had been talking to.

"That was Joanna," I said.

After Joanna and Andrea returned to New England, Mom asked me questions about Andrea. Who had been Andrea's boyfriend before she married her husband, John? I didn't know that there had been any prior boyfriend. As best I could, I reconstructed Andrea's life for Mom: Andrea had attended John Rennie High School in Quebec, had worked in Groton State Park in Vermont, and now she lived in Winsted, Connecticut, with John, having raised three children, several dogs and cats, and having turned their backyard into a virtual pet cemetery.

"I cannot imagine," she said, "how I could have lost the whole life of that little girl."

Mom was indignant the morning we picked up the hearing aid from Dr. Antonucci—the hearing aid Joanna paid for. It was a gloomy, rainy morning. Dr. Antonucci showed us how to maintain the hearing aid and offered a moisture-proof case for it for another eight dollars. I urged Mom to buy the case.

When we got back in the car to go home, Mom said, "That was so unfair of you. I cannot believe you would put me in that position."

She was livid that Dr. Antonucci would charge us eight dollars for a case moments after we had paid $2400 for the hearing aid. In principle, she had a point.

"Another thing I'll never forgive you for," Mom told me, "is the time I made cookies for you and brought a plate upstairs to your bedroom, and you and your friend were in there smoking pot."

I couldn't recall the incident with the plate of cookies, but it sounds like a likely story. She went on.

Harkening back to my arrival in June 2006 (it was now summer 2008), she told me that when I had first got there, I brought Jim Bouchard into their house and let him stay overnight without her and Daddy's permission.

Further, she said I had gone ahead and moved into the house on my own without talking to her and Daddy about it.

When Dr. Michael returned from Israel, I drove Mom over to his office. The gleaming black clearcoat on his BMW sports car was a refreshing sight. We waited for nearly an hour before he got to us. We sat in a small examining room with Mom wanting to discuss what could be done for Dad. Dr. Michael, though, was concerned about Mom's lack of concentration and her inability or unwillingness to answer his questions.

He ordered an immediate brain scan for Mom due to her "change in mental condition," so I drove her down the street to Radiology Associates to undergo the scan. It seemed like she had just had a brain scan the week before, but in any event, I left the office carrying a prior medical report that showed Mom had two stress fractures in her thoracic vertebrae.

There were moments in the never-ending debate about whether we could take care of Dad at home, moments when we were talked out, moments when no creative ideas could emerge, yet more continued to be said. I did not want a kleptomaniac home health professional staying in our house, sitting on the couch watching television, gutting the refrigerator; in Florida, these people were untrustworthy and prohibitively expensive.

One evening in the living room, the subject of taking care of Dad came up again, and I lost my composure.

I screamed, "I'm going to kill both of us!" before taking a seat on the couch in a state of exasperation and embarrassment.

Mom responded by patiently explaining that it was her and Dad's own fault that I was so emotional. As a child, I had had many problems, and they should have sought professional help for me then. Before it was too late, I thought.

Dad's wallet was missing. Mom had tucked it away for safe-keeping in a drawer of Dad's underwear and couldn't remember where it was. I thought Dad needed some kind of picture ID, so I drove him over to the VA outpatient hospital in New Port Richey. Using a VA wheelchair, Dad rolled up to the Admissions desk and proudly stated his name and social security number, beginning with "aught aught eight." At first the volunteer worker at Admissions had no idea what Dad meant.

After he had his picture taken and his new ID had been printed, Dad rolled over to the VA eye clinic to see if a doctor was available because he had missed his last appointment. There were no openings at the eye clinic, so we got back in the car and pulled out onto Little Road under a sky thick with clouds, a sky the color of a slab of marble.

As I drove north toward Windsor Woods, Dad made an excruciating request.

"Aren't you going to take me home, so I can see your mama?"

"We don't have time," I said. "I've got to get ready to go to work."

My words were spoken out of an instinct for self-preservation, or maybe out of selfishness or cowardice. I knew there was no wheelchair at home. I knew that the scene at Pineneedles Drive would be one of emotion and that extracting Dad from the home that he had not seen in weeks was guaranteed not to be easy.

"All right," Dad said, "I guess we don't have time."

He was making it easy for me. There was no way around it. Disregarding the wishes of my father, my grandparents, or my uncles, was an act of ingratitude and disrespect. My innards churned as I swung the Mercury up Fivay Road toward Dad's room at Windsor Woods.

Mom cracked her bedroom door and stuck her head out.

"Tell the others," she began, waving her fingers to indicate people, guests, daughters in particular, who must be dispersed about the house somewhere out of sight but not out of range of hearing. She had heard them talking and laughing.

I sometimes said, not to jar her, "Alright, thanks, Mom. I'll tell them."

Sometimes I turned my head to see her standing in the partly open door of the bedroom, her manner generous and vulnerable, and said to her, "Thanks, Mom, but no one's home now except the two of us."

I turned off the television and tried to imagine what Mom was experiencing in the world of her mixed dementia. It was unclear to me what to do. Andrea and I had tried to bring Mom's mental confusion to Dr. Michael's attention long ago. For instance, we tried to get him to write out a prognosis describing her mental confusion, but he had refused.

Now I wondered whether there was any basis in reality, any truth to the hallucinations that Mom saw and heard, something that ordinary perception was missing. Did we really know that her mother and Dad's great aunts did not visit our lawn and living room in some dreamy afterlife? Was I certain that, at the moment Mom heard my sisters' peals of laughter ring out, they were not in fact lifting a glass somewhere, partying with friends?

I listened for their laughter, their echo, without discernible result.

The golf course beckoned, and on Saturday mornings I followed, paying into the River Ridge men's scramble, usually winning back my entry fee. The third week in September, I started play on the back nine and had come around to the fourth hole on the front, the island hole that sat behind the row of houses on Baltusrol, across the street from the Keiths' house on Pineneedles. As I got up on the tee, hefted my pitching wedge, peered through the oak and cedar shadow over murky water swirled with pollen, I heard my mother's call for help like letters painted in the air. In the quiet surroundings of the tee box, I heard Mom in my intuition as clear as day.

I finished the last few holes, worrying. I drove home without going into the bar for a beer or waiting to hear what foursomes were in the money.

Although it was now twelve noon, Mom's bedroom door was closed. Without a doubt, something was wrong, and I felt a pang of guilt that I had not been there that morning.

I opened the door and called inside. Mom answered from her vanity, where she was seated on a chair with a towel bunched underneath her.

"Call an ambulance," she said. "I think I'm having a heart attack. I'm having chest pains."

I called the EMTs and went to help Mom. She couldn't get up. She had urinated on the folded towel. She had been calling for help when she saw the shadows of people passing on the street.

As the EMTs arrived, I felt embarrassed that I had reported a heart attack in progress, when apparently there was none. They asked me where I wanted Mom to be taken, and I told them Community Hospital, where Dad had been taken. I showered and got ready to go, heeding the EMTs advice not to rush.

"Oh, my God, how did you find me?" Mom said as I entered the hospital room.

Tests were done the next morning. Mom was upset, claiming that a "Chinaman" had raped her. That worried me, but I waited for Mom to say more about it, and later on, she recanted.

The tests revealed several problems, all difficult to isolate. Mom had a urinary tract infection. Her kidneys were not functioning properly, and there was a presence of cancer of undetermined location.

She stayed in Community Hospital for several days. It was obvious that she needed rehab to get her legs strong once again. I visited her at the hospital at noon, following the three-hour class I took at H&R Block. The CNAs found an extra lunch tray for me, so that week I ate pot roast and steak for lunch while keeping Mom company.

Mom tried to get out of bed, but the nurses didn't like it and fastened a strap across her stomach. I thought it was too tight, so I loosened it.

As Mom slept, I performed Reiki on her. At one point, she opened her eyes and said, "That's enough, now. They'll think you're in one of those clubs," referring to the Falun Gong.

The hospital staff seemed unaware of Mom's lactic intolerance, and her incontinence resurfaced She was greatly embarrassed by her incontinence, and as a solution she chose not eat.

"We could sell the house," Mom said. "We could move into one of the villas," she said, meaning the small homes along the sixth, seventh, and eighth holes at the golf course. "You could have a bedroom, and Daddy and I could have one. And you could stay there and teach at the school."

Knocked on her back, tired out from ailment and degeneration, Mom still tried to figure out where we should live.

I brought her handfuls of Tylenol, which she coveted. I bought her magazines from the gift shop, but the contents were really nothing but perfume ads. She requested, then insisted that I get her out of the hospital.

"I thought you would do me better than this," Mom said.

"Mom," I said, "I'm doing everything I can. If that's not good enough, then I'm terribly sorry."

After eating lunch in Mom's room at Community Hospital, I drove north on U.S. 19 to visit Dad at Windsor Woods.

SWALLOW STUDIES

———————— ❊ ————————

D ad didn't breathe a word of complaint about Windsor Woods. He wasn't a complainer. Dad had a roommate, briefly, a grouchy man who slept in the bed by the door. Once, the grouchy man grumbled something unpleasant to Mom, so I gave him the hex sign while he was sleeping. Soon after that, the man passed away.

Mom was appalled by my crossing my fingers over the guy's bed, but I told her that the guy had been grumpy to the wrong person. He deserved what he got.

The men at Windsor Woods were uprooted human beings, spending every moment on the brink of despair. All the precious hours they'd spent in quiet living rooms eating lunches carefully prepared by their wives, all those precious hours seemed somewhat wasted. All the grains of sand of late middle age had trickled through the glass, and no one could turn the glass over again. Nothing had prepared them for the shock of being institutionalized. They had hoped that the major battles of their lives had already been waged. Now they were being asked to summon the prodigious strength to rehabilitate.

I sat with Dad as he absorbed the news that Mom was in the hospital. A tattered and sun-bleached American flag hung not far from Dad's window rain or shine, night and day.

Dad told me that I had a lot on my plate now, visiting the two of them and taking care of the house. I gave him my progress report: I'd cleared the eaves and plugged armadillo dens around the foundation.

It was a little after three o'clock. The day was quieting down as most of the patients would be fed, washed and put in bed for the night before the nurses and CNAs changed shifts at four.

Dad sat in his wheelchair with his thin legs crossed and his long-nailed fingers interlaced.

"I'm supposed to go home in a few weeks," he said. Then he turned his palms upward and lifted his hands. "Unless that's just pie in the sky."

What might have provoked words of congratulations left me paralyzed. I couldn't say anything, not even a "That's good news, Dad." Absolutely nothing. I'd lost my ability to cope. I should have said something positive to Dad, at the same time knowing he would never come back home. I dreaded lifting, washing, caring for Dad.

Thus, when it was suggested that Dad could escape his confinement among the faded ocher walls and dingy tiled floors of Windsor Woods, I could not utter a syllable.

Marie, the occupational therapist, kept helping Dad like a woman on a mission. He sat and pronounced words as she listened and observed.

He swallowed pudding, put together puzzles, and importantly, enjoyed Marie's company. He'd been living on an Ensure diet for nearly three months. He negotiated the hallway with his walker, strapped to the physical therapist. Marie saw how hard Stephen was working.

Several women I'd seen visiting their husbands had been admitted as patients in Windsor Woods. The rehab would sustain them for a while, but none of them would again have the strength, balance, energy and mental clarity to live at home.

Now Mom needed rehab. I decided to admit Mom to Windsor Woods and put her in room 207—Dad's room, with Dad in his window bed and Mom in the bed by the door. I thought that Mom and Dad might derive some comfort from being together.

But this effort backfired. Her first day, Mom sat in her wheelchair calling the place a "dump" and stating to all who would listen, "We're only here for a little vacation. We're just here for a few days."

With Mom in the room, Dad became stricken with anxiety. He woke Mom up in the middle of the night, insisting that she start packing their clothes. As I appeared in the doorway of room 207, Dad rose out of his wheelchair and told me to get the car and bring it to the front of the building. Then I was supposed to get boxes and help them pack their clothes. They were both going home.

My heart sank. Mom could see the benumbed expression on my face.

From her wheelchair, she said, "What's the matter, Chris? I don't see that shine in your eyes today."

The pressure from Dad to take him home was reaching a peak. I had requested that a Hernando-Pasco Hospice nurse be assigned to evaluate Dad. A counselor and a Hospice nurse began to visit Dad each week.

Without trivializing her, let me say that the nurse, Kathy, was a "ten." An attractive blonde with a stunning body, she was pleasant to Dad and laughed at his jokes.

Kathy helped me out. I'd told her that I felt guilty about not taking care of Dad at home. I told her that Joann, our neighbor across the street, had exhorted me to bring Dad home. Kathy assured me that I was not capable of taking care of Dad by myself. He needed skilled nursing care. She said trying to care for him for at home would be the wrong thing to do. I was relieved and grateful for her involvement.

After being roused in the middle of the night by Dad, Mom was red-faced and tired. She refused to go into the physical therapy room. She slapped the wrists of the therapists.

"She hits," a female therapist told me.

I was alarmed that my gentle mother would have transformed into a strangely irrational creature hitting the people who were trying to help her—I was alarmed by the entire context. The staff moved Mom into another room up the hall so she could get away from Dad and get some rest at night.

She refused to start her physical therapy, so I had to convince her to begin. I advised Mom that Medicare would not pay for her stay if she didn't attend therapy sessions, and she would be thrown out.

"Hoo-ray!" she said, in defiance.

As the nurses put it, no one understands the stress level of a caretaker unless they see the patient every day. That's the only way to get the full picture, to get the full physical and psychological impact.

At one point, the Hospice counselor called to tell me that they were ending their visits to Dad since he was really in no danger. When I told them that Dad had fallen down in his room, though, they decided that the fall qualified him for Hospice care and that their visits would continue.

Fall was coming. My sisters had filled Mom's closet with slacks, jackets, sweaters, jerseys, sneakers. Mom ate her lunch in the dining room, a bustling but well-organized affair. I sat with Mom at lunchtime on many occasions. She ate little and invariably tried to give me her food. Many patients could not feed themselves, and the CNAs exercised their routines unfailingly, spooning mouthfuls of food into the patients, urging them to chew and to swallow.

I brought Mom her romance novels and puzzle books from home, but she didn't read the books or work on the puzzles. The books sat on a corner of her dresser, pushed out of the way. This was not a passing mood—this was a change in her state of being.

Anxiety coursed through both of them. Mom did not read; Dad didn't want to be read to. Prior to the crisis of his bleeding ulcer and his loss of blood, Dad could recite Macbeth's soliloquies in their entirety. Now he thought he slept in cellar holes.

I noticed that Mom wasn't wearing her hearing aid. The nurses were reluctant to let her wear the hearing aid, fearing that she would lose it. Without it, though, Mom was deaf. The acuity of her uncorrected ear was fifteen percent, so she needed the hearing aid in her corrected ear to know what was going on around her. I saw the hearing aid as a quality of life issue and pushed to initiate its use. I insisted that the nurses establish a routine for putting in Mom's hearing aid. Mom was much happier with it in. My own anxiety, though, greatly increased as Mom would tuck the hearing aid into hiding places where none of us could find it.

I talked with Dad in the car on the way back from Bayonet Point Regional Hospital where he had failed his swallow study.

"That's a kick in the head," Dad said.

"Dad," I said. "You really do have the choice. You could have the G-tube removed and eat regular food again if you wanted to."

After all, he had aspirated food for two years while living with me and Mom. The irony was that Dad had never been a voracious eater, except for desserts, and his Parkinson's disease had eliminated his sense of taste.

Now, though, Dad decided that he did not want to run the risk of choking to death. He decided to forgo dishes of ice cream with chocolate syrup and parfait glasses of butterscotch pudding for the safety of the feeding tube.

Mom developed an infection and was taken across the road to Bayonet Point Regional. At that point, my sister Andrea arrived, and we made the tandem visit first to Mom in the hospital and then to Dad in Windsor Woods.

In the hospital bed, Mom sat upright and told Andrea and me about a fight that had taken place downstairs in a post office which she believed was part of the hospital. She described a scene of great disruption, including the telling of falsehoods and the physical abuse of many people. As she told us about all the commotion, we could not begin to interrupt the momentum of her story-telling or to convince her that this big fight had been part of a dream.

Across the road at Windsor Woods, Dad told a tale of having seen in perfect detail a color guard of soldiers on parade. Andrea explained to Dad that since he was blind, had he seen all that detail, then he must have been dreaming.

Dad reported that the previous night he had been kept out on the lawn in a dog's cage.

HALLOWEEN, THANKSGIVING AND CHRISTMAS

———— ▪▫▪ ————

I hung Dad's plastic pumpkin lantern on the front porch.

I kept gas in both cars—my Nissan and Dad's Mercury. Every day I turned the ignition in one of the vehicles and set out in the direction of Windsor Woods, taking the back way out Osceola Road past corrals of horses standing in the shade of the oaks, past restored cars gleaming through plum-colored paint, past the shabby Elks Club and the nicotine-drenched VFW. Then for a couple of miles I flew down Fivay Road into a tunnel of 90-degree air flanked by walls of swaying green foliage. The ride was mesmerizing, and I noticed the change and felt nostalgic when fall came, burnishing the leaves and shrinking their volume.

I set up a haircut fund for Mom and Dad, and Dad got a haircut and Mom got her hair trimmed and styled every few weeks. Each of them looked a little embarrassed sitting in the stylist's chair, which was visible to people through a large panel of glass. The haircuts were important, though. They were about the only thing that gave Mom and Dad any pleasure.

One rainy day I met a young woman at Windsor Woods. I'd pushed Dad's wheelchair out to the screened-in porch and was telling him about how I had won money that morning even though the golf scramble had been rained out. The girl and her mother were on the porch trying to comfort the father, who was immobile and distressed, unable to talk.

We recognized some kinship in each other: people who were taking the time to be with men who had raised them, men who were not at the top of their game, men whose lives were like cities under the siege of artillery, or in my father's case, a U-boat being depth-charged.

We spoke in the hallway outside Dad's room. The girl was much taller than me. She was slim and attractive and had a gleam of intelligence in her eyes, or at least it seemed that way to me. She seemed to apprehend the urgency of the moment and to understand my need for communication.

I mentioned that our family was in the last stages of trying to qualify for assisted living in Connecticut and that we were going to give a final accounting of our finances to the assisted living facility that week.

"Don't give them a final accounting," she said. "Get an attorney."

She told me that I could save my parents' house from being gobbled up in the process. The girl's advice was for me to get Dad qualified for Medicaid to pay for his care in the nursing home. Besides, Florida has a homeowner policy that prevents the government from attaching the home to recoup the expenses which are covered by Medicaid. On the woman's advice, I got in touch with an attorney and began the process of qualifying both Mom and Dad for Medicaid, paying the fees out of their checking account.

Mom knew that she still had cash in the bank, of course. She had balanced the checkbook, or tried to, for years. Mom questioned me about money.

"Can't we go to the big bank some afternoon so I can take out some money?" she asked.

"I'm afraid that you'll lose the money," I said. "It's not advisable for any of the patients here to keep cash. Someone might take it. I've set up a fund for you in the office up front. For your haircuts or any other items you need."

She really wanted money, so I gave her a handful of one dollar bills which she kept in the pocket of her crocheted sweater.

I tried to save on the cost of hiring the wheelchair ambulance for Mom and Dad's doctor appointments, ferrying them back and forth myself. An oncologist had scheduled a bunch of appointments for Mom, but his office was located miles down U.S. 19 and all he did was draw her blood without publishing any results. I canceled as many appointments as feasible.

A month after Mom started living at Windsor Woods, Dad contracted pneumonia. He lay motionless in bed with the G-tube no longer attached. His breathing was laborious. The nurses administered antibiotics, but Dad's metabolism wasn't high enough for the antibiotics to work.

I hoped that Mom understood that Dad was ill. She wanted to go ask Dad about money. I wheeled her into room 207 and told her that Dad had pneumonia but offered no further postulation.

Tugging on his hand and wrist, she asked, "Daddy, do you remember how much money we had?"

Dad lay in bed, his rasping breath forced in and out.

"Well, we're not getting much out of him," Mom said.

She wheeled herself out of the room.

Later I checked on Dad. His eyes were open.

"Hi, Dad. It's Chris," I said.

"Well, Jesus Christ!" he exclaimed.

I could tell from his voice that he had been voyaging in nether regions, far from Windsor Woods, far from his son.

I had brought Dad an absentee ballot. When I asked Dad if he wanted to vote in the presidential election, he said, "No. I don't like either one of them. I hope they both lose."

Dad experienced a final evening of vigor, sitting up in his wheelchair, visiting with Mom in the lobby by the nurses' station. After this upsurge of energy, though, Dad would not get up again. Bare chested under his sheet, Dad was in the last hours of his long battle with glaucoma, diabetes, high blood pressure, and Parkinson's. His lungs were filling with fluid. He entered a state of terminal agitation, moving his limbs about constantly.

I stood in Dad's room with my back to the wire-reinforced window. Dad looked at me and reached out his hands, taking hold of my right arm. He pulled me toward him, and I leaned over the rail of the bed, succumbing to his grasp. I thought, maybe he wants to hug me one last time, but the expression on his face told me that something else was taking place. This wasn't a hug. I may have been a subject in a dream, a memory from Dad's days as a Vermont State Trooper. He held me with considerable strength, as if he were fighting to arrest a drunk.

I was alarmed that he was taking control of me—I feared being captured by the Senex and yanked into the realm of rigidity and death as if into a pit. I had to use a jujitsu to get out of Dad's grasp—following the limb downward to release the first hand and then circling my wrist to release the second. It was not a gentle action. A look of complete surprise overtook Dad's face as I broke his hold. I was free then, but guilt burrowed into me as I looked at Dad lying in his bed. I felt like I had rejected him.

Kathy, the Hospice nurse, called me one afternoon. She sounded distressed. She told me that Dad had developed tracheal congestion and was now in the process of dying. She gave him forty-eight hours. I emailed my sisters, telling them what Kathy had said. At Windsor Woods, I held my cell phone to Dad's ear as Joanna spoke to him, saying she was coming from Massachusetts to see him. Dad lived a couple days longer than Kathy's estimate, as if waiting for Joanna.

After Joanna arrived, I stayed at home for a couple days. I worked on stuff for school and let her drive to Windsor Woods and tend to the parents.

Tuesday night we got a call from the CNA on the night shift. Dad was dying, making crackling noises in his throat. Before we could get ready to drive to see him, we received another call—with the news that Dad had passed away.

Dad died at 12:30 a.m., Wednesday, October 29, 2008. The yellow wooden doors to the patient rooms in Dad's hall were closed. Dad lay shirtless in his bed with his mouth slightly opened. It was shocking to see him. I had the unmistakable feeling that Dad would sit up in bed and not die at all. I kissed his moist, cool forehead. I thanked the CNAs, Jody, a kind leprechaun, and Marie, a Hispanic girl, who had sat with Dad in his room while he died. Dad's angels.

It was heartening to learn the presence of a whole night shift I'd never met, people who knew Dad and enjoyed his sense of humor.

A man from North Meadowlawn came to take Dad's body. Joanna and I waited outside the room while the man prepared Dad to leave. A while later, by the van parked under the portico of Windsor Woods, in the timelessness of the middle of the night, I stood beside Dad and spoke to him until his body was loaded into the dark green van and he embarked on his last journey.

The following morning Joanna and I went over to Windsor Woods early to be sure we were the ones to tell Mom that Dad had died. Her room was across the hall and one door further down from what had been Dad's room.

She was sitting up on her bed, wearing her light slacks and sneakers, a white pullover, and an aqua-colored crocheted sweater. Joanna sat on the edge of the bed and told Mom that we had bad news and that Dad had passed away during the night.

"Oh, he did?" Mom said.

She cried, bearing the news of the death of her husband. News that was unfathomable to me.

The foolish hopes and dreams were spent: dreams of mine that Mom might survive Dad and live out an extended, socially-rewarding widowhood, smiling into advanced old age, taking phone calls from her grandchildren, dreams that were not to be.

The foolish hopes were gone. Mom now pushed and pedaled her wheelchair down the worn corridors of a nursing facility, learning the tiny pulling steps gripping with the balls of her feet, attempting to adhere to routine, the only course of action possible.

I was in a state of upheaval following Dad's death. Twice I lost my car keys, once on a cold night just before Thanksgiving. I'd locked myself out of my car at a 7-Eleven market and had to walk back to the house.

I had to skip visiting Mom for a day, and, the next day, when I entered her room just after lunch, her eyes were full of tears.

"Oh, God, I thought I'd lost you," she said.

The girls had visited Florida, she told me. They were here the entire weekend. Her daughters had visited Florida, but they had not come to see her.

"They were here, right out in the hallway. I could hear them," she said, "but they didn't come in. I can't imagine why they wouldn't come to see me."

I assured Mom that her daughters would have visited her, had they come to Florida. She must have been dreaming, I'd said, trying to comfort her.

Mom put on her windbreaker and large fashionable sunglasses, and I rolled her out into the fresh air of the yard and parked by a fence where we had our backs to the sun. She questioned me endlessly about money. She asked why we couldn't take one afternoon to drive to the bank, so she could get some money. The perennial question. I gave Mom another small roll of one-dollar bills which she tucked into her jacket pocket. I put her wheelchair into the trunk of the car and drove to Walgreen's and let Mom pick out nail polish and polish remover. The nurses took the bottles of solvent away from her, though, and kept them out of Mom's room.

The following week, I drove Mom out to Hudson Harbor to look at the water and the boats docked there in the cool perfect sunlight. I told her I was still looking for a nicer room for her, and it was true.

I arrived at Windsor Woods to find Mom in tears once again. With the shades open, the room was brightly lit. Mom was on her bed, propped up by pillows. A folded, brown shawl lay at the foot of the bed.

"Is anybody still alive?" Mom asked, circling her hands in an all-inclusive gesture.

"Yes," I said.

I named her daughters and their children, and Mom's nieces, Pammy and Susan.

"They are alive, and they think of you."

"I just want to go home," she said. "I want to go home and be with Mommy and Daddy and Uncle Charles, but I know it's impossible."

She yearned for the past of her childhood, for her own mother and brother and father, the father who'd worked as an engineer on the railroad and, every evening when he came home from work, had left hard candy in the pockets of his overcoat for her to find.

I felt her yearning for wholeness, simplicity, origin. I knew how impossible, how incomprehensible the nursing home was to her.

One day I came into the dining room and saw a man and two CNAs attempting to force food into Mom's mouth. I relieved them of their duty. I sat down beside Mom. When it was clear that she wasn't going to eat, I took her for a spin in her wheelchair. Whenever I took her out of her territory down the far wing of the nursing home, she wanted to go back to the area that she knew.

Mom was slowly pushing and pedaling past room 207 where Dad had lived and died. We turned to our right and looked into the room. Another man lay in the window bed looking the same way Dad had looked not long before his death, showing the same rugged yet shriveled profile, covered in a clean sheet.

Mom looked at the man and gestured toward him.

"Don't you wish that was *our* Daddy?" she asked.

We ate Thanksgiving dinner together at a table in the Windsor Woods dining room where a throng of people were visiting the residents. To be fair, it was an enjoyable turkey dinner with all the "fixin's."

As Christmas approached, I was concerned that Mom's door hadn't been decorated with paper bells and drawings the way other people's doors were. I brought in gift wrapping and cut it up and taped it to her door as a background. Diane, the head nurse, saw me doing this. I told her I just didn't want Mom to be overlooked. Diane assured me that Mom's door would be decorated like all the others, and on my next visit I saw that my crude efforts with the door had been replaced by a construction paper background and numerous cutout Christmas designs.

Turning to me from her bed, Mom said, "This is one of those years where we're just going to have to skip Christmas."

When someone survives their spouse's death in a nursing home, it's often advisable to move them, so they say. It's advisable to let them start afresh in another facility.

Early in December Joanna and I paid a visit to Trinity Rehab, a new nursing home only recently licensed to offer beds. Beds were available, the PR man wanted our business, and Joanna and I thought it was a no-brainer to get Mom into a larger, more modern facility.

Joanna had just left for New Hampshire when I got a call from Windsor Woods. Mom had fallen down in her room and struck her head on the bureau. As a consequence, Mom was being held down in her bed with restraining straps.

It was an overcast Thursday at lunchtime when I got to Windsor Woods. Mom was eating but not in the dining room. She sat at a table with several other patients in the occupational therapy kitchen. Therapists leaned over the patients offering them spoonfuls of mashed potatoes and gravy. Mom was winched into her wheelchair. I made room for myself next to Mom.

The moment I sat down, Mom told me, "I can't do this anymore."

I loosened the belt that held Mom in her chair.

"I'm getting you out of here," I said. "I've got a room for you."

"Thank God," Mom said. "I can't thank you enough."

"You don't have to be here any longer, Mom," I said. "We're moving you today."

We left the eating therapy session and went back to Mom's room.

Mom laid back and rested on her bed as I procured boxes and packed her belongings. December was windy and cool now, and her closet was filled with clothing. Mom had every type of slipper, pullover, sweater, slack, windbreaker, and piece of workout gear. Mom's transfer was due to take place at three o'clock that afternoon.

The room was packed up, and it was time to prepare Mom for the trip. Her hearing aid had to be taken out and recorded as a separate item and placed into the care of the ambulance driver who would transport Mom to Trinity. The CNA told me she needed my help as Mom wouldn't remove her hearing aid. Mom said it wasn't necessary to take out the hearing aid, and she turned her head away from me on her pillow and pretended to sleep.

For the safe keeping of the hearing aid, I told Mom, it needed to be carried by the driver. Again, Mom said she wasn't going to take it out, and she turned her head aside and feinted an instant state of deep sleep.

I stated as many times as it took, with no invested emotion, that Mom needed to give me her hearing aid. At last, she raised her head, removed it from her left ear, and handed it to me. I gave it to the CNA who put it in its box.

A nurse joined us, and as the nurse and the CNA got Mom ready, Mom told them that she did not want to leave; instead, she wanted to stay here at Windsor Woods. They reported this to me, and I did not say anything. In the same breath, Mom had told the nurse she wanted me to get out of her room. Thus informed, I went outside, crossed under an oak tree in the haze of the parking lot and drove home.

I arrived at Trinity the next morning. Mom was sitting in the corridor in her wheelchair. When she saw me, she said, "I don't know if they have a room for me."

I said, "Of course, they do. Let's go look at your room."

She had a double room and a spacious bath to herself. Everything in the room was brand new. No one had ever slept in the bed. The bath robes were thick terrycloth with Trinity logos.

My worry was the absence of the nurses Mom had known at Windsor Woods, the absence of the familiar environment. The comfort of Trinity's living room was unmatched, yet the patients were too weak and disorganized to enjoy the common rooms. Nobody sat on the couches;

nobody watched the large screen TV.

And the staff was sparse—only one CNA on Mom's floor and one nurse behind a huge horseshoe workstation with six or seven incapacitated adults sitting in wheelchairs nearby. From a sophisticated, aged face among the row of wheelchairs came a scream of discontent and indignation. From the dark of a room came another patient's repeated call for "nurse, nurse, nurse."

After golf on Saturday morning, I dropped in on Mom and found her asleep in her bed, so I left with intentions of visiting longer on Sunday.

Sunday morning I worked at the laptop computer entering grades into an electronic grade book. The school semester was over. All I had to was calculate all the grades and submit them online. So I arrived at Trinity a little past noon on Sunday.

I twice walked past Mom in the hall before asking the Asian nurse who was on duty, "Where is Barbara Keith?"

"She's right there," she said.

I looked at the row of people crumpled into their wheelchairs. One of them was Mom, slumped over with her head almost touching her chest.

"Mom," I said. "Are you all right?"

She was trying to wipe drool from her mouth with the sleeve of her turquoise sweater.

She uttered what I thought was, "Thank God it's you," or "Thanks to you."

I was not sure exactly what she said. I told the nurse that something was wrong with my mother. This was not the demeanor or posture she had maintained at any point in her life. I'd never seen her like this. She had to go back into her room immediately. The nurse complied. When

Mom was laid down, she fell unconscious.

The nurse tried to reassure me saying, "See, she's comfortably resting now."

I asked if Mom had eaten anything at breakfast that morning. Not a bite. I inquired as to what medications she was being given. Only half an Oxycontin—nothing from the list of medications she had been taking at Windsor Woods was being administered. I didn't see a glass of water nearby.

The nurse called the on-call doctor who turned out to be Dr. Sheila Drevon, Dad's former doctor. The nurse gave the vital signs to Dr. Drevon over the phone. Dr. Drevon recommended that Mom be taken to an emergency room for observation. I told them to take Mom to Bayonet Point Regional, which was across Fivay Road from Windsor Woods.

I sat with Mom in the emergency room at Bayonet Point in the afternoon. She was unconscious and pale. Mom had a severe urinary tract infection. At dinnertime, I drove home and ate, then drove back to the hospital. At eight o'clock that night Mom was wheeled upstairs to a room. The male nurse who admitted Mom to her room showed me deep bedsores on Mom's butt to be sure I knew about them. He promised to treat them and assured me they would heal.

On Monday a cute and energetic nurse attended to Mom. I had started taking a morning class in tax preparation, so I spent the afternoon studying in Mom's room. I expressed concern over Mom and asked the nurse if Mom was going to pass away.

"No, she's not going to die," she said, in a chiding manner.

In the meantime, on the elevator in Bayonet Regional, I ran into one of the administrators from Windsor Woods. He asked about Mom, and I told him that Mom was upstairs and was sick.

Tuesday, there was a "no feeding" sign on Mom's door. Like Dad, she had lost her ability to swallow safely, according to the medical staff. Mom had come back to consciousness somewhat. She tried to talk to me nearly nonstop, but I could not make out a word she was saying. There was congestion in her throat. Mary Keith, who was working her volunteer shift, came into the room and saw Mom. Mom saw Mary and spoke quite a few sentences to her, but her language was incomprehensible.

As she left, Mary turned to me and said, "She's not doing very well."

I was quite concerned because shortly after the tracheal congestion developed in Dad, he had died. And Mom was showing the impatient physical movement that Kathy, the Hospice nurse, had called terminal agitation. At the end of the day, having listened to Mom explaining something I could not make out and having the feeling that I was missing out on vital instructions which could be Mom's final ones, I got ready to go home for the night.

Mom looked at me with frustration and exclaimed, "Is that how you're going to do it? Do you want me to get mad at you!"

And she sat up and began to tear off her nightgown.

On Wednesday, Dr. Talwar, a doctor of Indian descent, called me and asked my permission to insert a feeding tube through Mom's nose into her stomach. Reluctantly, I consented, hoping that Mom could be kept alive long enough for her to regain some strength. The procedure took several hours, and when I visited Mom in her room, her hands were tied to the bed rails with restraints because she wanted to pull the tube out of her nose.

It was nine o'clock Wednesday night. I leaned against the wall of the corridor outside Mom's room and waited for what seemed like forever until the tall, Jewish nurse checked on all the patients and updated their charts. From what I had gathered, this nurse was one of senior members of the nursing staff. I asked her what she thought the prognosis was for Mom.

"We'll just have to wait and see," was her response as she made some notations on her chart.

The nurses either did not want to or did not know how to talk about death and dying. It seemed to me that when someone is close to dying, that's the time to show all your cards, to say whatever you have to say to help anybody involved.

In the meantime I received a message from Trinity Rehab notifying me that, in the event Mom was discharged from Bayonet Point Regional, they could not readmit her.

As I took a shower Thursday morning, I realized there was no more time to waste. The tracheal congestion was a clear sign that Mom was dying. I called the hospital and spoke with their resident Hospice nurse. Within minutes the Hospice nurse called me back and said that, indeed, Mom was a candidate for Hospice. I asked her what I had to do, and the Hospice nurse said she would take care of everything. We arranged to transfer Mom to the Hospice on Rowan Road in New Port Richey. Again, Mom would be transported at three o'clock. Taking the POA and Mom's living will with me, I drove to Bayonet Point and waited with Mom in her room until just prior to her transport, then I drove to Hospice and admitted Mom.

As soon as Mom was placed in the bed at Hospice, she opened her eyes.

"Well, hello," I heard the nurses say to Mom. "Chris is here."

When the nurses pulled the feeding tube out of Mom's nose, she reacted with a flinch.

It was December 18. In the soft light of the hallway outside Mom's room stood a lovely Christmas tree decorated with lights and gold ribbon.

"You're in Hospice, Mom," I said, "and you finally have a nice room."

I had brought Mom's Bible, a gift from her mother and father. I read aloud the nativity stories from the Gospels, the accounts of travel, the search for a place to stay. I read the Twenty-Third Psalm, Mom's favorite, and I read other Psalms that contained the language of weaponry and war.

I took my tax exam the following morning. I arrived at Hospice at two o'clock on Friday afternoon. Mom was awake, and I read her some short poems by Wordsworth and Yeats. Then I read Mom several pages from Alice Walker's story, "Everyday Use," about the family quilts and the rivalry of the two daughters. It was a sunny afternoon. The room was bright and quiet. Mom was looking at me and paying attention to the reading. Although her hair was whitish gray now, she had always been a redhead, and there was an amber coloration to her brown eyes.

As I read to her, I sat by the side of the bed with my back to the windows. Her face was to my left, her head supported by pillows. As I read, Mom's eyes brightened, and the amber color became pronounced. Rays of amber light flickered and shot out of her eyes past my shoulder. The effect was so clear that I stopped reading for a second, asking myself, "What was that?"

By then, Mom had done a yeoman's job of paying attention. I didn't want to carry on too long. As I brought the reading to a close, Mom looked at me and spoke the first half of a syllable, "eh," and I felt that I knew in its entirety what she intended to say, what a well-written story by Alice Walker.

As I stood up to take a seat on the couch across the room, I saw that Mom's eyes had closed halfway and looked dull. She breathed quietly, and I moved my hand back and forth in her field of vision to see if she would react, but she did not.

At seven-thirty, Mom's eyes remained half-closed, yet she quietly breathed. I made the decision to go home and get ready for a job interview scheduled for the next morning. At nine o'clock that same evening, I was on the telephone with Joanna. Joanna was telling me that she had just called Hospice and requested that Mom's phone be held up to her ear. The nurse had put the phone up to Mom's ear, but Joanna had heard footsteps walking away and felt that no one was there. While I was speaking to Joanna, Hospice called my cell phone to tell me that Mom had stopped breathing.

An ornament in the shape of a lacy angel hung on Mom's door. I cried when I saw her. I cried in relief that Mom's struggles were over. I cried in gratitude that Hospice had had a room for Mom where she could have peace and dignity as she passed from this world.

The driver came from North Meadowlawn. He appeared burdened with distress, looking down at the floor and wiping his forehead as he came down the carpeted hallway. I told him I remembered him, as he was the same man who had picked up Dad after he died at Windsor Woods.

When all was prepared, he opened the French doors which led from

Mom's room to the cool night outside, and between the room and the night there was no division at all, the air flowed in, and the two of us pushed the gurney bearing Mom's body down the strip of sidewalk to where the van awaited. As the van pulled away and turned down Rowan Road, Mom began her journey into the afterlife, but first she would follow Dad, only fifty-one days behind him, through the fiery portal of North Meadowlawn.

PITHLACHASCOTEE RIVER

————◆————

From its headwaters at Crews Lake, the Pithlachascotee River wends its way southward through pine flats and grassland, cuts through palmetto forest in the northwest corner of Starkey Wilderness Preserve, and courses toward the Gulf of Mexico where it broadens and endures the back and forth wash of the tide. In downtown New Port Richey the surface of the blackwater river looks like a smooth sheet of black plastic. As its waters merge with Millers Bayou, its surface turns blue.

Time passes and things in the world undergo their transformations. The pride of my father, an association called the U.S. Submarine Veterans of World War II, founded in 1955, lost its federal charter and was decommissioned in 2010. Its members have vanished. Recently I saw an old man wearing a USS *Gar* baseball hat being helped by his son at the door of the dentist office. I held the door for them. I couldn't resist telling the son that my father, too, had served in the Silent Service during the War in the Pacific. As he got his father through the door, the son listed off all the war patrols his father had been on.

Back in the day, Dad used to jitterbug with my mother and roll her over his back and swung her in the air—during his days in the Navy—feats that seemed unthinkable. Now Mom and Dad have been laid to rest.

Today, a younger vet who served in the Gulf War lives in the house on the double lot on the corner of Baltusrol and Pineneedles. Most people at River Ridge don't remember Dad, but there are some who do. Some of Mom's friends are still alive; Mrs. Nagy went so far as to visit Mom at Windsor Woods. I imagine that that visit took some guts and compassion to complete. She even invited me to come over for a drink, but I haven't gone.

Mom and Dad are like ghosts in the neighborhood of Pineneedles Drive. Lost to the awareness of people living there now.

It is a willful and conscious decision to exercise patience with someone who needs help. We all have limits, but they can be vastly expanded through our willfulness. During my childhood, my relationship with my mother was at times not a sweet story, although I later trusted her and turned to her for advice throughout my adult life. As for Dad, he kept to himself a great deal, and as a kid, I found it difficult to make much of an impression on him. We did not enjoy the camaraderie of classic father-to-son ties, if such ties even exist.

It's understandable that some people cannot take care of their parents. It's not a mortal sin or a moral failure if you cannot help, to my way of thinking.

The tall lady I met at Windsor Woods told me that each person has their special gift to share. We each make our contribution. She said this to me in a precious timeless conversation in the hallway of a nursing home. It was something I needed to hear. I hope to say something like that to you, too, through this story.

Years ago I could not imagine my parents passing from this world, and I couldn't imagine this backdrop: a city full of people on the fringes of society, the motorcycles and muscle cars, the people out walking their dogs and thinking of those friends and neighbors who have passed before them, the cry of the hawk, the vast migrations of the crows, the sliding along of the tannin-rich blackwater river, the Boat Building River.

I'm grateful that for the last sixteen years of their lives Mom and Dad lived in their quiet neighborhood in Tall Pines. They went about their routines, took their pleasure cruises while they were able, came home and played cards with neighbors, discussed their worries, followed the football games.

No one can entirely be spared from harm, but I do wish good health and longevity to the elder citizens of our country. I have seen courage in their faces when there is nothing left for esteem to draw on.

I close with gratitude that the Starkey Wilderness Preserve wrapped around their neighborhood, providing for them a lush quietude, keeping all its creatures, and my parents, too, safe in the palmetto cradle.

REFLECTION

After my parents died, the holidays passed, and I let things resonate around me. I sat in the screened-in porch and watched deer moving silently in the dusk, cutting through our hedge only a few feet from my chair.

Friends happened to stay with me for a couple of weeks. They were traveling to their house in the Caribbean from visiting their son and his family up north. They told me to start taking down some of my parents' furnishings and to remodel a little to make the house feel more like my own. I pulled the curtains back from all the glass doors giving the house an open feel.

After they first passed away, I felt relief as if a goal had been achieved. Mom and Dad had journeyed all the way to their deaths, a journey that we, too, will take in our own time. We may wish the end of our own lives would be somehow easier in comparison, but there's no guarantee.

Numbness alternated with a state of amazement. Longer-lasting grief did not set in until I sold my parents' house and moved out.

It was upsetting to disgorge the houseful of my parents' things. I was fascinated by all the parfait dishes and cake pedestals and seasonal items they possessed. I made up thirteen boxes of "surprise packages" containing bourbon and shot glasses, vases and butter dishes, candle holders and similar items, and taped them closed and included them in an estate sale. The surprise packages sold like hotcakes.

I hired a probate attorney and petitioned for an Order of Summary Administration to take care of my mother's estate.

Phone calls had come pouring in after Dad passed away. More calls and emails came in when Mom died just before Christmas. Some of these phone conversations had a ring of finality to them, like I could tell I wasn't going to continue to get more calls of support from these same people. They'd played their roles in supporting me as I was supporting Mom and Dad in the nursing home and hospitals. I'm sure some of them had experienced a lot of emotion through their conversations with me, and now they had to turn their focus to their own families.

Selling the house brought out the worst in me emotionally. I was anxious. I made mistakes such as tearing down hard window dressings and throwing them in the dump, only to find out that that wasn't what the realtor meant by "cleaning the place out." In fact, the window dressings were specifically mentioned in the P&S Agreement, but I hadn't read the P&S carefully enough. Frankly, I didn't know what I was doing and didn't have anyone there keeping me in line, saying things like, "Hey, what are doing? Leave that window dressing alone!"

The aftermath gave me occasion to vent emotion and come apart somewhat in a way that I didn't have leisure to do when Mom and Dad needed me.

Yes, I drank five cups of coffee and tore up $600 of custom fixtures, only to wake up crying the next morning after I realized what I had done.

I filled the armadillo holes around the house, had the stucco painted with Elastomeric to conceal the cracks, had the Yucca trees in the back yard removed. We shipped the Hitchcock entertainment center and my Grandmother Moore's bureau up to Connecticut. My nephews took the USS *Ray*'s battle flag which had hung in Dad's bedroom.

I moved out of 10435 Pineneedles Drive to a little place on Tennessee Alley in the poorer section of town. I took Mom's orchids with me and burned a couple of them by leaving them out in the hot April sunshine. Late in the mornings, I went swimming at the aquatic center nearby. Then I took forty-five minute naps every afternoon, falling into delicious oblivion.

I had an apartment full of cleansers, jars of screws and bolts that Dad had collected, piles of towels from Mom's closets, enough Oxiclean to last a lifetime. I had the bedroom set from my room at Mom and Dad's, and I had their tube television. It was a low budget operation.

I also had a towel rack on wheels that I put in the hall outside my bathroom. I'd found the rack in Mom's roomy, bedroom closet. Whenever I went in and out of the bathroom in my apartment and glanced at that towel rack, my eyes teared up.

I was amazed that my parents had lived and had gone away. Living in the same house with them again had been an amazing experience. I felt like the secret to life was right in my fingers if I could just see it for what it was.

When I thought of my mother's ordeal of taking care of Dad and managing every bill that came into the house and ordering all the medication, I sobbed for minutes at a time.

Hernando-Pasco Hospice offered grief counseling to all family members, if people wanted it. I gave them $800 of what had originally been Dad's money as a thank-you for their palliative care of Mom. I even considered meeting a counselor at Hospice, but I was hesitant to do so and determined to manage on my own.

In fact, I was worried that I was experiencing profound grief, so called, until I read the detailed description: people who had profound grief sometimes stopped going out, stopped eating, stopped laughing.

Living with my mother and father meant learning not to show false pride. One noticeable change in me, undeniably, is that I came away from the experience with a heightened respect for elderly people.

"Life doesn't end on a high note," reads a line from one of my journals. It's amazing to me that the great moments of people's lives, the fun, the drama, what they lived through, just aren't visible to us as we glance at the elderly. Most of their finest chapters are far behind them. We don't give the elderly much credit because we can't see into their lives the way we should be able to. We're a selfish, ageist culture. We owe people respect.

I had other new feelings. Besides a respect for the elderly, I had a new openness to and interest in children. I liked going to the laundromat and watching the Mexican children as they played, glimpsing their shining black hair and darkly gleaming eyes, none of the children crying out in protest, none of them upset, sprawling on the laundromat floor like lost socks.

My original plan had been to keep Mom and Dad in their house as long as possible. Our family had waited too long to start coping with the onset of their old age. My parents were hard to manage and didn't invite our suggestions. As a result, living in a skilled nursing home turned out to be a shock to them. They never had a chance to adjust to the nursing home because by the time they went in, it shocked them into a state of denial.

I have read that 81% of cases of dementia go undiagnosed. In my mother's case, my sister and I tried to get Dr. Michael to pay attention to Mom's mental confusion, but he did not respond like that issue had urgency. There is always a question of how to manage multiple regimens, that is, different maladies or diseases at the same time. I had hoped to get Mom to reduce the laundry list of medications she was taking. In fact, Andrea commented that Mom was self-diagnosing at certain points over the years.

Once Mom entered the nursing home, the jolt from normal reality was complete. Dad, though, suffered a post-op delirium, basically transforming overnight from a cynical bright older man to a bewildered, anxious person struck down with physical injury and on the verge of capitulating to parkinsonism.

Having seen my mother and father pass away, fifty-two days apart, my most basic thought is this: death is natural and normal. When the body wears out, when the body's metabolism is so slow that medicine cannot help the person, it is time to die.

As sad as it may be to the survivors, given our connection to them, it is unfair to ask them to live a single day longer.

My close friend tells me that she felt orphaned after her mother passed away and after her father needed to be admitted to an Alzheimer's unit. Taking care of her parents had become life's structure for her. She felt the loss of the two people who had given her unconditional love.

I came to the conclusion that there is nothing on this earth more important that a person can do than to help someone who is dying: someone vulnerable, someone drawing on their last resources of strength, someone who cannot do things on their own, someone possibly disoriented, sometimes fearful.

If you have helped someone in this way, my message is that you have done something important, something meaningful, for the world. I hope you find an inner nourishment from your experience and especially realize that although what you did may have been an extenuated inconvenient way to live for a while, helping another person in their moment of need is what you were supposed to be doing. Nothing could be more important.

Within my family, it was quite hard to discuss private issues and concerns. Many times Mom and Dad told me to stay out of a certain problem. It was an uphill battle to give them guidance because they were inured to being in charge.

I am so grateful for those of you who fight for the dignity of another person, when their powers of influence are at a low.

If given the chance to do some of this over again, I wouldn't allow the doctor to insert a feeding tube into my mother only a few days prior to her death. I would listen to my inner voice that told me she was ready to die. I would have saved her hours of unnecessary discomfort.

But I didn't know then what I know now.

My parents showed their character and their lack of bitterness through how they faced the end of their lives.

I will never forget Mom looking into Dad's room at Windsor Woods, after Dad had passed away, seeing the man with craggy features draped in a white sheet, lying in what had been Dad's bed. She turned to me, saying, "Don't you wish that was *our* Daddy?"

Even though Dad was struggling near his end, Mom would have rather had him living. She loved him that much. Even on the worn linoleum tiles of a nursing home, no one was hastening this world to its end.

Mom and Dad. Although none of us predicted the rapid onset of the end of their lives, their spirits were courageous and their actions were worthy.

ABOUT THE
AUTHOR

Christopher Keith, a former karate instructor and composition teacher, has also published *Introduction to Asian Long Staff Fighting*, a martial arts DVD and workbook, and *Headhunter: The Blues Odyssey of J.D. Nicholson*, the oral history of an influential West Coast blues piano player. He is now at work on *Posh Corps: Peace Corps Philippines*, a memoir, as well as *Tennessee Alley*, a collection of fiction. Previously, he studied creative writing with Raymond Carver at Syracuse University in the 1980s and earned an M.A. from the Writing Program.

www.ingramcontent.com/pod-product-compliance
Lightning Source LLC
Chambersburg PA
CBHW051913170526
45168CB00001B/361